Groups in
Health Care Settings

The *Social Work with Groups* series

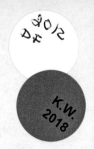

Groups in Health Care Settings

Janice H. Schopler
Maeda J. Galinsky
Editors

The Haworth Press
New York • London

Groups in Health Care Settings has also been published as *Social Work with Groups*, Volume 12, Number 4 1989.

The Haworth Press, Inc., 10 Alice Street, Binghamton, NY 13904-1580
EUROSPAN/Haworth, 3 Henrietta Street, London WC2E 8LU England

Library of Congress Cataloging-in-Publication Data

Groups in health care settings / Janice H. Schopler, Maeda J. Galinsky, editors.
    p. cm.
    "Has also been published as Social work with groups, volume 12, number 4, 1989" — T.p. verso.
    Includes bibliographical references.
    ISBN 0-86656-972-3 : $29.95. — ISBN 0-86656-973-1 (pbk.)
    1. Medical social work — United States. 2. Social group work — United States. 3. Self-help groups — United States. I. Schopler, Janice J. II. Galinsky, Maeda J.
    [DNLM: 1. Group Processes. 2. Health Services. 3. Self-Help Groups. 4. Social Environment. 5. Social Work — methods. W1S0137MB v. 12 no. 4 / W 322 G882]
HV687.5.U5G76 1990
362.1'0425 — dc20
DNLM/DLC
for Library of Congress   90-4018
                                                           CIP

Groups in Health Care Settings

CONTENTS

ABOUT THE EDITORS

Janice H. Schopler, PhD, MSW, is Associate Professor at the School of Social Work, University of North Carolina at Chapel Hill. She earned her master's degree at the University of Michigan in Ann Arbor. Her doctorate is in health policy and administration from the School of Public Health at the University of North Carolina at Chapel Hill.

Maeda J. Galinsky, PhD, MSW, is Professor at the School of Social Work, University of North Carolina at Chapel Hill. She earned her master's degree and her doctorate in social work and psychology at the University of Michigan, Ann Arbor.

Drs. Schopler and Galinsky have published numerous articles and chapters related to their group work research, practice, and teaching. Their emphasis has been on providing group leaders with theoretical frameworks and practical guidelines for their practice. They have been active in testing established theory, evaluating interventions and practice outcomes, and describing and conceptualizing innovative forms of group work practice. They are most widely cited for their work on goals, co-leadership, potential dangers of groups, and open-ended groups. Both editors consult frequently with social workers and other professionals about groups in hospitals and other health settings and have a particular interest in the ways groups can be used for education, support, and treatment in health settings.

Groups in
Health Care Settings

Preface

The social consequences of illness for patients and their loved ones are widely recognized as a significant aspect of health care. Social workers have long understood this and, since the early decades of the century, have sought the establishment of their professional services in hospitals, clinics and agencies serving health needs, in order to strengthen the care of ill people and to enhance their getting and remaining well.

The group work component of social work practice has had only a peripheral place in the institutionalized acceptance of the profession in the health care system. However, as with all health and mental health services, the power of interpersonal relations and social well-being that the small group can make possible in the process of healing and sustaining health has been growing in recognition.

This volume, so knowledgeably edited by Drs. Janice Schopler and Maeda Galinsky, testifies to the relevance of group life and social group work practice in the countering of fragmentation and non-holistic tendencies in today's medical care. It also testifies to the venturesomeness of social work staff in health institutions and agencies — and their colleagues in medicine, nursing and administration — who believe in the generative qualities in the group.

Realistically the volume suggests the unevenness of the acceptance of social group work as an important adjunct to medical care. For example, we note the absence of program activity. The inability of group workers to employ expressive activities, non-verbal exercises, and the full panoply of "the doing" of group life points to the tentativeness of social group work in medical and health settings, and symbolizes the certainty that the method has not yet been able to make its fullest contribution.

We can predict that the presence of social work with groups in the health care system will continue to expand as the commitment to

xiii

holistic thinking further embues the medical establishment. We can also predict that social workers who understand the group method will persist in contributing to the advance of a holistic conception of health care through the creativity and humanness of their practice model.

We warmly congratulate Drs. Schopler and Galinsky on the insights of their introduction and the distinguished quality of their selections and design for this volume dedicated to social group with practice in health care.

Catherine P. Papell
Beulah Rothman
Editors, Social Work with Groups

Introduction:
Social Group Work:
Promoting a More Holistic Approach
to Health Care

Janice H. Schopler
Maeda J. Galinsky

As medical treatments grow more complicated and the health care system increases in complexity, patient care can become fragmented and impersonal. Although advances in medical technology and increased efficiency in the delivery of services are associated with more positive physical prognoses and improved quality of care, they can also lead to a widening gap between the health care providers and recipients of service. Social workers have often attempted to fill that gap by giving personal attention to the social and psychic needs that typically accompany biological distress. Social group work is, by no means, a complete antidote to forces that depersonalize and frustrate patients and their families and put pressure on staff, but groups can be used to promote a more holistic approach to health care and the promotion of health.

Although social workers have been using groups in health care settings since the turn of the century, groups have often been a relatively marginal service in a system that favors one-to-one intervention. In recent years, the profusion of publications related to groups in health care suggests a marked increase in the use of this approach (e.g., Berkman, Bonander, Kemler, Marcus, Rubinger,

---

Janice H. Schopler, PhD, and Maeda J. Galinsky, PhD, are affiliated with the School of Social Work, University of North Carolina, 223 E. Franklin Street, CB #3550, Chapel Hill, NC 27599-3550.

1

Rutchick, & Silverman, 1988; Carlton, 1986; Getzel, 1986; Lonergan, 1985; Northen, 1983). Several factors may have prompted the resurgence of interest in social group work services in health settings during the past decade. Certainly, the group method has potential for building mutual aid systems and for mediating between the individual and the often confusing maze of health care services. Groups can be an effective, time-saving way to convey information and build support systems. Groups also are viewed as a cost effective means of providing service to a greater number of patients and their families. The expanding literature on the versatility and benefits of health care groups is encouraging, but many articles also speak to existing barriers to implementing group services in health care systems. *Groups in Health Care Settings* focuses on many ways that social workers can use groups to facilitate a more humanistic response to the needs of consumers and providers and addresses the skills that are needed to gain institutional support for group services in health care systems.

The lead article by Helen Northen provides the framework for understanding current social work practice with groups in health care. Her scholarly review of 244 publications points to the practical ways groups are being used to enhance "feelings of intimacy and connectedness that offset the experiences of isolation and helplessness" in health care. Northen also identifies limitations in the literature: reports of group work with children, adolescents and the elderly are sparse; structured activities are seldom used to achieve group purposes; the impact of ethnic and religious values on the use of groups and medical services is often overlooked; and, the interface of group services with other systems receives little attention. The review concludes with an affirmation of the progress made in the past decade in work with groups in health care settings. Based on her assessment of the literature, Northen issues the following challenges to social workers: address the limitations in the current literature; collaborate with other health care professionals to assure accessibility, continuity and comprehensiveness of health care; and, promote the development of groups in health care through research related to planning, intervention, and outcomes. With this volume, we begin to respond to these challenges.

As Helen Northen notes, disease and health crises are often the common denominators that draw participants in health care groups together. The need for versatility in structuring groups in health settings stems from the wide range of diseases and health conditions, the different requirements of inpatient, outpatient, and community settings, and the varied needs and concerns of the diverse participants. In this volume, the articles address groups related to such major health concerns as heart disease, cancer, AIDS, sickle cell disease, life threatening health crises, and terminal conditions. The groups meet in hospitals, clinics, and the community and tend to have flexible boundaries with open admission of new members or short term member commitments. Participants include patients, family members, significant others, and staff. The recurrent purposes include: support, education, information, training, problem-solving, and empowerment.

Despite the diversity of these articles, several strong themes emerge: (1) members can be helpful to each other when they recognize their commonalities; (2) support and self-help groups that convey information, teach skills, and create a network of supportive bonds can be a force for empowerment; (3) the impact of the context of service must be considered; (4) responsiveness to cultural factors stemming from differences in race, ethnicity, and economic status is critical to positive group interaction; (5) the evaluation of interventions and outcomes as well as the development of relevant theory are critical to the development of groups in health care settings.

The articles by Gilbert and by Abramson deal with the organizational context of service. Gilbert discusses the factors to consider in implementing group work service in health care settings. The theoretical framework she provides is illustrated with examples from her experience in developing a mothers group on the pediatric ward of a large hospital and offers practical guidance about how to gain institutional acceptance and support for a group program. Abramson addresses the way social workers can use their group work skills to influence the operation of health care teams responsible for coordinating patient care. Her exploration of the social worker's pivotal role on health care teams draws on literature related to social group work, interdisciplinary teams, and consultation, as well as her own experience. After identifying barriers that often interfere with effective teamwork, Abramson proposes and illustrates strategies that social workers can use to enhance team operation in their roles as team members, leaders, and consultants.

The remaining articles detail the ways in which members come together in groups focused on their common health concerns. Patients, family members, and significant others offer support and assistance to each other in these groups. Group sessions empower their members by offering them an opportunity to share their experiences and fears, gain information, consider new approaches to their problems, and develop skills for dealing with illness, the health care system, and the community. Social workers serve in a variety of capacities, sometimes taking responsibility for leadership and, at other times, facilitating the self-help orientation of the group. Empowerment tends to be a dominant theme, whether explicitly stated or implicitly assumed.

Several of the articles describe the way groups can benefit members with a common disease. Child and Getzel describe a group approach to "rebuilding the shattered identities of inner city persons with AIDS" and utilize case illustrations to highlight strategies for dealing with group issues. Nash, reporting results from his survey of self-help groups for individuals with sickle cell anemia and their families, stresses the empowering force of the support, education, networking, and advocacy these groups offer their members. Subramanian and Ell focus on the use of groups to help low income Black, Hispanic, and Anglo patients cope with a first heart attack. Their model is based on their critical assessment of the needs of this population for coping skills and social support.

Other articles discuss the way groups can be helpful to relatives and staff members who are close to patients who have similar conditions or who are experiencing similar health crises. Chesney, Rounds, and Chesler evaluate self-help groups for parents of children with cancer and identify factors related to group structure, professional involvement, group activities, and parent characteristics that increase the value these groups have for members. Holmes-Garrett describes the way social workers can use single session groups to respond to the needs of relatives of patients in the intensive care unit for information, guidance, and support. Bauman and James also recognize the critical roles relatives can play in patient care and recovery. They discuss a support group for families of burn patients that has evolved from clinical experience as well as their survey of the literature and practitioners in similar settings. Finally, Richman reports survey results that indicate the multiple functions groups are serving for clients and team members in hospice settings and gives particular emphasis to the way staff support groups can reduce stress and enhance patient care.

The articles in this special volume exemplify many of the creative approaches that practitioners and researchers are taking to advance the development of groups and promote more holistic health care. The predominant focus is on adult groups whose members come together and are empowered through the process of sharing mutual concerns, gaining helpful information, developing coping skills and reaching out to each other with care and support. The authors tend to build on existing theory and knowledge and provide practical guidance for dealing with the health care system and guiding group interaction. Several pay particular attention to ethnic and cultural factors in designing group interventions. None of the articles relate to groups for children, adolescents or the elderly. Furthermore, the use of structured exercises is rarely discussed as a way to promote goal achievement. These omissions suggest an agenda for the future. The articles included in this volume are, however, characteristic of the varied roles social workers are assuming in promoting support and self-help groups and advance our understanding of how groups can facilitate more caring, responsive delivery of health services.

REFERENCES

Berkman, B., Bonander, E., Kemler, B., Marcus, L., Rubinger, M.I., Rutchick, I., & Silverman, P. (1988). Group work practice in health care. In *Social work in health care: A review of the literature* (pp. 21-34). Chicago: American Hospital Association.

Carlton, T.O. (1986, Summer). Group process and group work in health social work practice. *Social Work with Groups, 9*(2), 5-20.

Getzel, G.S. (1986). Social work groups in health settings: Four emerging approaches. *Social Work in Health Care, 12*(1), 23-38.

Lonergan, E.C. (1985). *Group intervention: How to begin and maintain groups in medical and psychiatric settings*. New York: Jason Aronson.

Northen, H. (1983). Social work groups in health settings: Promises and problems. *Social Work in Health Care, 8*(3), 107-121.

Social Work Practice
with Groups in Health Care

Helen Northen

SUMMARY. A survey of 244 publications attests to the burgeoning interest in groups of patients and families as an important modality of practice in health settings. Therapy groups predominate, followed in frequency by groups for purposes of support, education, crisis resolution, socialization, training, and mediation. A biopsychosocial theoretical orientation provides the foundation knowledge used by a large majority of authors. The rationale for using groups is clearly related to the problems faced by clients, combined with understanding how to mobilize the therapeutic forces that operate in groups. Important limitations in the content of the literature are identified, including a need for research on process and outcome.

TRENDS IN THE LITERATURE

From the earliest days of social work practice, some farsighted planners in both medicine and social work recognized the value of groups in meeting the needs of patients. In one of the very first books on social work, Ida Cannon set forth principles of diagnosis and treatment, recognizing that social workers needed to work with patients, their families, and groups of patients (Cannon, 1913, 1923). The first group therapy had been used at Massachusetts General Hospital in 1905 with patients suffering from tuberculosis. That was in the days before distinctions were made between social casework and social group work as separate methods. For a variety of

---

Helen Northen, PhD, is Professor Emeritus, School of Social Work, University of Southern California at Los Angeles.

Address correspondence to the author at 2311 Chambers Lace Drive, SE, Lacey, WA 98503.

reasons, interest in work with individuals and work with groups soon diverged and work with family units was almost forgotten. In the field of health, social workers virtually became caseworkers helping individuals one by one. But gradually, beginning in the 1940s, hospital personnel began to recognize the value of groups, particularly on children's wards and in Army and Veterans Administration hospitals.

By 1959, interest in groups in the field of health had advanced enough for the National Association of Social Workers to appoint a committee to study the use of groups in health settings and to identify issues that would warrant further study. Based on the work of the committee, the first book on the use of groups in health settings was published, with Louise Frey (1966) as editor. The bibliography listed twenty-three articles that described group work in health care. By far, the greatest number were about services to children, either on pediatric wards or in community agencies serving physically handicapped people. Only three articles dealt with adult patients, one with ward living, and one with the social worker as member of an interdisciplinary team. Two were general articles that described the roles of group workers in hospitals. The division between group work and casework was clearly evident.

There has been a rapid increase in the literature on groups in health care, particularly since 1975. A survey of literature conducted during the preparation of this article, identified 244 publications on social work practice with groups in the field of health. The scope of the survey was limited to general works and to articles about groups of patients and members of their families which were co-led or led by a social worker. It did not include the large number of self-help and support groups that do not use the services of professionals. The material was published in numerous journals and edited books. Most of the references consist primarily of descriptions of single groups dealing with a particular illness or disability and a few deal with hospitalization, terminal illness, chronic pain, loss and mourning, or death. Some forms of illness have dominated the literature. Groups of cancer patients or their families are by far the most frequently described (40 articles). Next in frequency were physical disabilities (16), kidney disease (10), Alzheimers disease and related dementias (9), epilepsy (7), and visual impairment (6).

There are one or more articles on almost every known medical condition covering a total of 32 different diseases or disabilities. Several publications deal with generic knowledge, skills, and issues related to the use of groups in health settings, including one book on the subject (Lonergan, 1982).

Numerous authors reported some form of evaluation of outcomes, usually through the use of follow-up questionnaires completed by members or based on worker judgments. Only two articles reported evaluation of the effectiveness of the group experience based on controlled experimental research (Subramanian and Rose, 1985; Subramanian, 1986). One other article described the use of a quasi-experimental comparative design to test the effectiveness of groups in training students in the health professions (Berkman and Rutchick, 1987).

There is a strong trend toward work with groups of adults, which represent 70 percent of all publications. Some readers may regret that social workers have not continued to take leadership in the provision of services to children and adolescents, as they did prior to Frey's summary. Only 19 articles were devoted to groups of children and 7 more to adolescents (11 percent of the total) and, only 18 articles (7 percent) focused on groups to meet the needs of elderly patients or their caretakers. The remaining publications were general and not age specific.

Another major trend is toward the use of verbal means for helping people. Very little attention in the recent literature is given to the use of activity-oriented experiences: talk predominates.

RATIONALE FOR GROUPS

The literature on use of groups as well as evidence from research attests to the need for practitioners to attend to the emotional, psychological, and social determinants and consequences of illness and disability. Group experiences can be helpful in meeting the psychosocial needs of patients and their relatives in many ways. All people need to develop and sustain satisfying connections with other people; human relatedness is the key to healthy development and functioning. The fact that people need people is the raison d'etre for using planned group experiences to help patients and their families to deal with the emotional stress and socio-emotional problems that accompany a severe illness or disability.

A medical illness or disability upsets the patient's steady state, disrupting interpersonal relationships, and changing patterns of role functioning. The illness or handicap of one person requires shifts in the attitudes, role expectations, and behavior of all concerned; it requires complementary adaptations by other family members, colleagues, friends, and others. These other people may support or sabotage realistic adaptation to the medical situation. The stress created by the illness is aggravated when other problems exist in the family, in friendships, or at work or school. Groups have special values in helping clients and their families to cope with the emotional distress and changes in living occasioned by the medical event.

There is considerable agreement that the therapeutic group mechanisms of mutual support and mutual stimulation are especially pertinent to work in the field of health (e.g., Boyd, 1977; Northen, 1983). The literature describes how the group process is well suited to ameliorating the emotional stress felt by many patients and their families who have feelings of isolation, loneliness, guilt, stigmatization, depression, helplessness, or hopelessness. In a successful group, these feelings are counteracted by a sense of belonging to a group in which a person feels understood and accepted, a powerful dynamic in the process of change.

As members of a group universalize their experiences, they perceive that they are no longer unique and alone. Since the group's purpose is one of enhancement or betterment, it is implied that members are expected to move toward physical and social health. As they come in contact with other members who are coping successfully with some problems, they develop a sense of hopefulness to replace the earlier one of uncertainty or hopelessness. Many patients and their relatives lack supportive sanction for ventilating the flow of feelings and painful experiences that accompany illness and its aftermath. The group provides a safe and supportive milieu for this important step toward channeling affect constructively. As accurate information is provided by the practitioner or knowledgeable members, myths and erroneous beliefs are eliminated. Distorted perceptions or ineffective behaviors are challenged through the interactional process in the group, which becomes a medium for testing reality. The group provides a reference outside the family against which to measure and judge one's own thoughts and actions. The group thus serves as a corrective for distorted perceptions and relationships. The multiplicity of reactions and viewpoints provide the person with feedback relating to particular interpersonal needs or life issues.

The therapeutic mechanisms that operate in social work groups are clearly relevant to work with patients and their relatives – therapeutic corrective relationships, mutual support, acceptance, universalization, instillation of hope, altruism, acquisition of knowledge and skills, catharsis, reality testing, and appropriate expectations (Boyd, 1977; Northen, 1988; Roback, 1984; Yalom, 1970, 1975, 1985). The particular forces that operate vary with the group's purposes, structure, and content.

PURPOSES OF GROUPS

The major purposes for which groups are used in health care are several: (1) provide peer support in relieving the inevitable stress felt by patients and families in facing and dealing with the illness or disability; (2) provide essential knowledge and skills pertinent to the medical condition and to changes in social living; (3) help patients and families resolve crises; (4) help patients and families to change or improve in some aspects of their psychosocial functioning that interfere with their social relationships; and (5) resolve interpersonal conflicts.

Several types of groups are described in the literature – therapy, support, education, multiple family, crisis intervention, socialization, training, mediation, and discharge planning. A large majority of the groups are composed of patients, but with some trend toward groups for relatives or other caretakers. The authors' own statements about types of groups were used to classify articles on health care groups. When an author did not name the type, the designation was given according to an analysis of the major goals of the group. There is considerable overlapping in purposes, and readers might differ on the assignment of a particular group to a category. Table 1

Table 1

Classification of Articles by Group Type and Composition

	Patients	Relatives	Both	Other	Total	%
Therapy	75	15	11		101	41.4
Support	25	38	2		65	26.6
Education	15	9	2		26	10.7
Crisis Int.	3	4			7	2.9
Socialization	7				7	2.9
Training				4	4	1.6
Mediation	3				3	1.2
Discharge Plan	1				1	.4
Sub total	129	66	15	4	214	87.7
General					30	12.3
Total					244	100.0

summarizes the articles related to groups in health settings by type of groups and population served.

General publications go beyond description of particular groups or programs to general descriptions of the use of groups in health care and summaries of selected samples of the literature.

Therapy Groups

Therapeutic groups predominate in the social work literature (e.g., Coven, 1981; Krausz, 1980). The general purpose of such groups is to help members identify and change aspects of psychosocial and family functioning that are interfering with the progress of patients or family members toward health. The need for therapy relates to knowledge that the normal interpersonal relationships of patients, families, and others have been disrupted by the medical condition or premorbid problems have been aggravated by the illness or disability. The goals of therapy go beyond support, reduction of anxiety, education, and provision of practical resources. They may be to: resolve problems in communication and relationships; increase capacity to face, understand, and manage the emotional reactions to serious illness and its threats to loss and death; help members to adapt to new roles or changes in expectations; and understand and correct distortions in perceptions of reality.

Certain common themes are discussed in therapeutic groups, regardless of the specific illness or disability. These include: (1) the impact of illness or disability on the patient and family; (2) ventilation and understanding the sources of feelings and behavioral reactions; (3) difficulties in interpersonal relations; (4) managing the pain, discomfort, and loss of functioning caused by medical treatment; (5) decision-making, including identification and selection of options; (6) clarifying the reality of situations and one's part in them; and (7) exploring, understanding, and changing maladaptive responses.

Although some therapy groups are open-ended, a majority tend to be semi-closed, admitting new members only at certain times, usually when a vacancy occurs. Generally the groups have a flexible structure, with formal roles limited to those of member and practitioner who engage primarily in expressive, exploratory, reflective, and problem-solving discussions. Some groups are planned, short-term ones lasting for eight to fourteen sessions; others are long-term or continuous groups with gradual changes in membership. Members usually meet once a week for between one and two hours. Often, however, members contact each other between meetings, developing a social network that continues after termination. These contacts provide reciprocal support and diminish the sense of isolation.

Selection of members is often based on a pre-group interview to assess the prospective members' desire and suitability for the group, or it is based on referral made by members of the treatment team. Groups are generally homogeneous in terms of type of illness or disability and stage of the life cycle, but heterogeneous in other respects. Sharing a particular medical condition creates a strong enough bond to make other differences less important than in some other fields of practice.

One important subgroup of articles on group therapy, eleven in number, are those composed of two or more families or subsystems of families, sometimes classified separately as multiple family or couple therapy (e.g., D'Affeitte and Weitz, 1974; Stainglass et al., 1982). Such groups combine the advantages of group and family therapy, offering support, challenge, and new ideas from peers as well as family members. Across family influences and cross-inter-action from family to family can be effective in shaking up rigid norms or patterns of communication, or bringing new information into each family. In essence, a culture is created that frees family members to face, in the safety of the group, what they might not have been able to face within their own family, for example, the reality of the fatal illness of a child.

The major goals of these groups are to involve the family in the patient's treatment; to improve communication between genera-tions; to clarify role expectations and make necessary changes in roles; and to resolve problems in interpersonal and intrafamily rela-tionships. The focus is on both each family and the interaction among families.

In other settings, multiple family therapy groups usually deal with whole family units including children, but this is seldom true in the field of health. The predominant pattern noted in the literature was groups of several couples, ill members and spouses. In other instances, the families consisted of the patient and whatever family members were available, with only an occasional mix of parents and children. As in other groups, the tendency is to place families with patients having the same medical problem in a group. Most groups have co-leaders and are either open-ended or closed short-term services, with no predominant pattern emerging. The term family is used inconsistently, often to mean simply that a group is open to anyone in the patient's family who chooses to come.

Support Groups

The provision of support is a major focus of most types of groups, but many groups have it as their major purpose (Appalone, 1978; Carey and Hanse, 1985). A support group is an aggregate of persons who have a common concern and come together to support and aid one another in coping with certain stresses and difficulties.

In health, the common concern is an illness, disability, or death. The use of professional leadership for support groups is a recent phenomenon.

All people need a network of supportive social relationships for satisfactory living, particularly important in patients' efforts to cope with stress occasioned by the medical event. But support is often withheld. Other people may be threatened and made uncomfortable by the patient's condition, particularly when the disease is a life threatening, contagious, or stigmatizing one. Dunkel-Schetter and Wortman (1982, pp. 70-71) give evidence that the more unfortunate the plight or the greater the distress, the more threatened, uncomfortable, and rejecting other people tend to become. Those most in need of formal support are less likely to receive it. Thus, groups become an important form of social support.

The need for professional leadership comes from the realization that peers do not always qualify as effective providers of support. Left to their own devices, groups can be unhelpful (Galinsky and Schopler, 1977). The feelings, problems, and experiences that members present are often distressing and complex. There is a fine line between the needs for education, support, or therapy. Natural helpers may or may not be equipped to respond appropriately to the needs of patients or families of patients who are severely ill or undergoing frightening and uncertain treatment (Blythe, 1983). Even when there are other sources of support, social work groups combine support with other healing mechanisms and focus on the achievement of goals particularly relevant to clients' needs.

The goals of support groups usually include one or more of the following: to reduce stress and social isolation; to enhance capacity to cope with diagnoses, hospitalization, and treatment regimens; to generate a sense of belonging; to provide opportunities for ventilation and universalization of feelings and concerns; to provide opportunities for socializing with persons with whom one has something in common; to enhance self-esteem and lessen feelings of being stigmatized; and, to learn about the medical condition and its treatment and about available resources in the hospital and community. As with therapy groups, specific goals vary with the nature of the group and the needs of its members.

Support groups tend to be structured with a clear focus and pre-planned content, education about the medical situation, ventilation of feelings, use of resources, and ways of coping. Co-leadership with a nurse is most frequent. The social worker usually directs the meeting with the co-leader being responsible for the medical aspects of the presentations or discussions. The groups vary in size, sometimes being larger than what are considered to be small groups. They are typically open-ended, with members coming as often as they choose, and with frequent shifts in self-selected membership. The focus of the group sessions tends to be on the content and in some instances, on the relationships and interactions among the members.

Education — Psychoeducation

Formal and informal groups are organized to impart knowledge and develop competence in areas of common interest to their members (e.g., Dooley, Prochaska, and Klibanoff, 1983; Pueschel and Yeatman, 1977). The purpose of educational groups in health care is to help patients or members of their families learn about hospitalization, medical personnel, available resources, and an illness or disability — its etiology, course, and consequences for personal and social living. A related purpose is to learn specific skills relevant to the patient's care. Education supports medical treatment and reduces stress and uncertainty through the provision of necessary information by experts. Some groups are small, closed groups, but most of them are open to anyone and sometimes last for only a single session.

In psychoeducational groups, the emphasis goes beyond didactic presentations, discussion, and teaching of skills to helping the members to express and understand their reactions to the content and the implications of the material for them, through the use of group process-oriented discussions. These groups are typically semi-closed in order to make possible the acquisition of knowledge and skills in a brief six to eight week period. Most are co-led, with a nurse or physician along with a social worker. A majority of groups are composed of patients, but some are organized for members of their families or for both patients and relatives. The medical situations and populations for which these different groups are formed are varied; for example, parents of high risk infants, children with cancer or other serious diseases, women receiving abortions or hysterectomies, older men preparing to move into a nursing facility, men with juvenile diabetes, and young adult blind people.

Educational groups perform an important function when they are adapted to the particular needs of the members. As knowledge and skills of group process are used, there is peer support and stimulation to assimilate and discover the applicability of the information to the members' situations. People often perform more effectively if they have knowledge and know what is desirable or effective in coping with an illness or disability. They may need new information or reinforcement of knowledge in order to make social decisions about themselves and other persons who are significant to them. Since emotions and relationships can obscure educational messages, members can benefit from discussions that help them to bridge the cognitive and affective aspects of learning.

Crisis Intervention

Several articles deal with the purpose of helping patients, and often members of their families, to move toward resolution of a particular crisis (e.g., Bergen, 1984; Spink, 1976). Crisis intervention has been defined as "a process for actively influencing the psychosocial functioning of individuals, families, and small groups during a period of acute disequilibrium" (Parad, Selby, and Quinlan, 1976, p. 305). The normal problem-solving processes have become immobilized. The major purpose is to restore social functioning. Goals usually include: (1) to cushion the impact of a stressful event through group support; (2) to enable clients to mobilize and use their capacities and resources for adaptive coping with the effects of stress; (3) to prevent damaging consequences of unresolved crises. To achieve these goals, early access to help is essential.

There is considerable confusion in the use of the term crisis in the literature. A large majority of the articles use the word "crises," but often this is in reference to an event such as an accident or diagnosis, rather than to the upset in the patient's or family's steady state. Thus, workers may not apply what is known about crisis intervention in their work.

The state of crisis is brought about by a precipitating event which is stressful. The same event may be extremely stressful for some people and not for others. When people become upset, there are marked symptoms of distress and distortions in behaving, feeling, and thinking. Coping capacities are overburdened. The crisis state is thought to be time limited, as is intervention.

Crisis intervention should be an important form of group services within the health field because many patients and/or their families are in a state of crisis. The articles on crisis intervention deal with crises occasioned by hospitalization, surgery, diagnoses of a severe illness, treatment procedures that fail, or death. In health settings, the typical short-term treatment is often modified. When working with patients with feared, life threatening illnesses, such as AIDS and cancer, periodic crises arise within the ongoing therapeutic group (Lopez and Getzel, 1984). As persons adapt successfully in one crisis situation, they may be more likely to deal effectively with subsequent ones.

Socialization

The category of socialization groups is a broad and general one, consisting of articles that describe groups of children and adolescents and adult patients needing long-term care (e.g., Eisenstein, 1959; Young, 1957). The purposes of socialization groups are to provide opportunities for social learning, developing competence in new roles or changes in roles in novel situations. According to Hartford, the goals of socialization are self-development of the members and enhancement of role performance or provision of compensatory opportunities (Hartford, 1971). These goals are particularly applicable in health settings where patients are often faced with making major changes in self perception and social expectations.

Young people enter hospitals with many fears and uncertainties about life in the hospital and diagnostic and treatment procedures. They are separated from family, friends, and familiar environments. They often feel isolated and alone, lacking normal opportunities for daily living and relationships with peers. In a group, they have the opportunity to express positive and negative feelings and learn that these are accepted and understood; they may secure medical information suited to their readiness to assimilate it which reduces the frightening quality of the unknown; they may participate in activities that compensate to some extent for the loss of normal channels of activities; they may find supportive relationships with other children and practitioners; and they may use play and other activities to work out their concerns and anxieties about the medical condition and treatment.

Most groups are open to all patients within reasonable age ranges. Membership in a group may be very short-term but intensive members may participate in discussions which are interspersed with activities. Some groups, particularly when hospitalization or rehabilitation is long term, are organized as clubs, allowing for maximum participation in planning and conducting the program.

Other Groups

A few articles included descriptions of other types of groups. It was surprising to find few cases in which the primary purpose of the group was mediation (e.g., Lipton and Malter, 1971; Weiner, 1959). In such groups, the goals are to help members to take major responsibility, to negotiate conflict between patients and staff, and to modify staff's dysfunctional attitudes and behavior toward patients. In other types of groups, it is an ongoing part of a social worker's responsibility to deal with such environmental obstacles. Several articles describe the use of groups for purposes of training nurses, physicians, and other health care personnel (e.g., Beckerman, 1987; Gaumont and Durock, 1980). Only one article presents the use of groups for purposes of discharge planning (Dougherty, 1982).

GENERAL PUBLICATIONS

In addition to the works that describe a particular group or program of groups, others deal with more generic conceptualizations of practice or issues. Lonergan's book on social work with groups in medical and psychiatric settings is a major addition to the literature (Lonergan, 1982). Several articles have surveyed samples of the literature (Carlton, 1986; Getzel, 1986; Gitterman, 1982; Northen, 1983; Olson, 1986; Rosenberg and Neill, 1982) beginning with the previously mentioned monograph edited by Frey (1966). Other writers have summarized the literature on particular diseases: Busch (1984) on group therapy with residents of nursing homes; Galinsky (1985) on groups for cancer patients and their families; and Hartford and Parson (1982) on groups for relatives of dependent older adults. Numerous other articles describe and assess the use of groups in the field of health.

The Content of the Literature

Certain content occurs over and over again in the literature. The literature generally describes the use of groups with patients and/or their relatives who are coping with stresses related to the psychosocial aspects of a particular disease or disability. Increasingly, the rationale for use of groups is quite clear, tied to understanding of the potentially therapeutic forces that operate in groups as these interlock with the needs of clients. Formulations of group purposes are similar to those presented in this article. Several writers report the need to translate the general purposes into more specific objectives that are derived from an assessment of psychosocial needs and matching needs to services. Most articles give some attention to pre-group planning and describe the formation, composition, and structure of the group. Many groups make use of co-leadership, frequently a social worker with a nurse or physician. Verbal presentations and interaction predominate: very little use is made of action-oriented experiences. Most articles present the themes that comprise the content of the group experience, a number of which are common across disease entities. They include sharing of experiences about the medical situation; offering expressions of support; ventilation of feelings; securing information; sharing ideas about how to cope with stress and particular problems; and, when the disease is life threatening, existential considerations of facing the issue of life and death.

Several writers (e.g., Lonergan, 1980; Gitterman, 1982) are concerned that too little attention is given to the social context of service. In spite of a strong emphasis on social as well as psychological and biological facets of illness and disability, little attention is given to cultural factors related to race, ethnicity, religious beliefs, and economic status. Further, only limited consideration is given to gaining adequate sanction from administrators and other personnel. Unless a plan for a group is carefully made and negotiated with significant other persons, there is little chance of success. There must be clarity about how the group experience will benefit the patients and the hospital and how it will be coordinated with other components of the patient's treatment and daily living.

A small number of articles deal in depth with group development and the use of group process. Since mutual support and mutual aid are essential to the group's effectiveness, more attention needs to be given to the complexity of group relationships and interactions and the ways practitioners facilitate the process to advance movement toward individual and group goals.

Work with groups of seriously ill or dying patients is bound to create stress for practitioners, engendering many powerful emotions of anxiety, guilt, depression, or helplessness. The complexity of group relationships and interactions creates challenges to competent practice. Workers may become overwhelmed by the multiplicity and intensity of feelings that are ventilated in the group. They may over-identify with some especially needy persons or take sides with patients against their families or medical personnel. They may avoid freeing the group to deal with powerful material or feel greater empathy with some than with other patients. They may not be able to respond therapeutically when members project their own anger and frustration onto them. They may have their own belief systems challenged when persons with whom they have invested great efforts get worse or die. When the needs of members are great, they may be tempted to deal with members one by one, but they will not be effective unless they can find the common ground that underlies the apparently chaotic diversity.

Several publications addressed countertransference in terms of the impact of group issues on practitioners. The feelings and problems of members may stir up unresolved personal issues in the practitioner's past or present. Workers' reactions to members may then be based on misperceptions of reality. Practitioners need to find time to reflect on their own feelings and reactions toward the group and to find support and aid from colleagues or supervisors in order to manage the feelings that are bound to occur.

A THEORETICAL BASE EMERGES

It is surprising, perhaps, that few clear differences in theoretical orientations to practice are evident in the literature. Knowledge about the interrelation of biological, psychological, and social aspects of health and illness has been accelerating rapidly and provides the foundation knowledge used by a large majority of authors in describing their work with groups. This summary substantiates Getzel's (1986) findings that there is a growing commitment to biopsychosocial models of assessment and intervention. What comes through clearly is the overwhelming need to attend to the strong emotional responses to illness and disability and to help clients to recognize, accept, and deal with them. Affect, as well as cognition and behavior, needs attention. The concepts of stress, crisis, coping, adaptation, and problem-solving are used repeatedly. Clear also is the necessity to understand the particular clinical manifestations of the disease or disability and its impact on patient, family, and significant other persons. What is not clearly integrated into the biopsychosocial base is the effect of environmental, including cultural, factors on the medical situation and on social work intervention.

The second major theoretical base is small group theory. Considerable attention is given to the values of groups and to social relationships as a key to healthy physical, emotional, and social development. Traditional definitions of groups, however, have been extended and adapted to the special nature of practice in medical settings. Brief service and open-ended groups may be more like aggregates of people than small groups. In such situations, the focus of practice tends to be less on the development of a cohesive group in which the dynamic healing forces operate most fully and more on meeting the immediate needs of the members. This observation is consistent with one of Gitterman's (1982) conclusions that group development has been neglected and with Olson's (1986) concern that too little attention is given to the workers' roles in facilitating mutual aid and recognizing and managing differences and conflict. Some recent articles (e.g., Lubell, 1986; White and Baker, 1977) integrate the biopyschosocial framework with theory concerning the development of groups and their processes. Further work on such integration is a task for the future.

Upon completing the review of the literature, there emerged an overwhelming sense of agreement with Mervis (1983, p. 128) that work with groups in health care settings can provide "life sustaining opportunities by restoring feelings of intimacy and connectedness that offset the experiences of isolation and helplessness." There was also a sense of satisfaction that progress has been made during this decade. Although most of the articles are descriptions of particular groups, the authors generally analyze the relevant knowledge and skills. It is clear that most practice is based on knowledge about emotional, behavioral, and social consequences of illness and disability for patients and their families. The rationale for the use of groups is clearly related to the difficulties faced by clients, combined with knowledge that the dynamic forces that operate in groups are well suited to meeting client needs. The biopsychosocial framework is translated into skills in assessment, pre-planning of groups, and intervention in group relationships and group interaction within stages of group development.

Reviewing the past has been exciting but planning for the future is a challenge; much work needs to be done. Several major limitations in the content of the literature need to be addressed: the relative neglect of work with children, adolescents, and elderly adults; inadequate attention to the selective use of activity-oriented experiences to further group proposes; and a serious omission of ethnic-religious values and traditions that influence the use of groups and medical care in general. Groups are often described as though they are the sole service provided, without consideration of the impact of the group on families and other social systems and of how group work supplements or complements other health and social services. Accessibility, continuity, and comprehensiveness of care are principles that are sometimes violated. Group work cannot go it alone; workers need to collaborate as team members to assure that the principles are followed. Finally, it is obvious that the time has come for research on practice with groups in health settings—research on planning and interventive skills as well as on outcome.

REFERENCES

Appalone, C. (1978, Winter). Preventive social work intervention with families of children with epilepsy. *Social Work in Health Care, 4*(2), 139-148.

Beckerman, A.H. (1987). Group work and medical education. In J. Lassner, K. Powell, & E. Finnegan (Eds.), *Social group work: Competence and values in practice* (pp. 209-221). New York: The Haworth Press.

Berger, J. (1984, Winter). Crisis intervention: A drop-in support group for cancer patients and their families. *Social Work in Health Care, 10*(2), 81-92.

Berkman, B. & Rutchick, I. (1987, May). Improving the sensitivity of health professionals to the needs of patients and families: An experiment. *Small Group Behavior, 18*(2), 239-53.

Blythe, B.J. (1983). Social support networks in health care and health promotion. In J.K. Whittaker & J. Garbarino. *Social support networks: Informal helping in the social services* (pp. 107-31). New York: Aldine.

Boyd, R.R. (1977). Developing new norms for parents of fatally ill children to facilitate coping. In E.R. Prichard (Ed.), *Social work with the dying patient and the family* (pp. 251-65). New York: Columbia University Press.

Busch, C.D. (1984). Common themes in group psychotherapy with older adult nursing home residents: A review of selected literature. *Clinical Gerontologist, 2*(3), 25-38.

Cannon, I.M. (1913, 1923). *Social work in hospitals*. New York: Russel Sage Foundation.

Carey, B. & Hanse, S. (1985-86, Winter). Social work groups with institutionalized Alzheimer disease victims. *Journal of Gerontological Social Work, 9*(2), 15-25.

Carlton, T.O. (1986, Summer). Group process and group work in health social work practice. *Social Work with Groups, 9*(2), 5-20.

Coven, C.R. (1981). Ongoing group treatment with severely disturbed medical outpatients: The formation process. *International Journal of Group Psychotherapy, 31*(1), 99-116.

D'Afflitti, J. & Weitz, G.W. (1974). Rehabilitating the stroke patient through patient-family groups. *International Journal of Group Psychotherapy, 25*(3), 323-332.

Dooley, B., Prochaska, J., & Klibanoff, P. (1983). What next: An educational program for parents of newborns. *Social Work in Health Care, 8*(4), 85-104.

Dougherty, H. (1982). Social group work in health settings: A discharge planning group for orthopedic patients and a therapeutic community for problem drinkers. In A. Lurie, G. Rosenberg, & S. Pinsky (Eds.), *Social Work with Groups in Health Settings*. New York: Prodist.

Dunkel-Schetter, C. & Wortman, C.B. (1982). The interpersonal dynamics of cancer: Problems in social relationships and their impact on the patient. In H.S. Friedman & M.R. DiMatteo (Eds.), *Interpersonal issues in health care* (pp. 69-100). New York: Academic Press.

Eisenstein, F. (1959). Life enrichment of the seriously handicapped through the group work process. *Social Work with Groups, 1959* (pp. 30-40). New York: National Association of Social Workers.

Frey, L.R. (Ed.). (1966). *Use of Groups in the Health Field*. New York: National Association of Social Workers.

Galinsky, M.J. (1985). Groups for cancer patients and their families: Purposes and group conditions. In M. Sundel, P. Glasser, R. Sarri, & R. Vinter (Eds.), *Individual change through small groups* (2nd Ed.). New York: Free Press.

Galinsky, M.J. & Schopler, J.H. (1977, March). Warning: Groups may be dangerous. *Social Work, 22*(2), 89-94.

Gaumont, B. & Dworak, M. (1980, August). Group work with nurses. *Health and Social Work, 9*(3), 71-77.

Getzel, G.S. (1986). Social work groups in health settings: Four emerging approaches. *Social Work in Health Care, 12*(1), 23-38.

Gitterman, A. (1982). The use of groups in health settings. In A. Levy, G. Rosenberg, & S. Pinsky (Eds.), *Social work with groups in health settings* (pp. 6-24). New York: Prodist.

Hartford, M.E. (1971). *Groups in social work*. New York: Columbia University Press.

Hartford, M.E. & Parson, R. (1982, Summer). Use of groups with relatives of dependent older adults. *Social Work with Groups, 5*(2), 77-89.

Krausz, S.L. (1980). Group psychotherapy with legally blind patients. *Clinical Social Work Journal, 8*(1), 37-49.

Lipton, H. & Malter, S. (1971). The social worker as mediator on a hospital ward. In S. Schwartz & S.R. Zalba (Eds.), *The practice of group work*. New York: Columbia University Press.

Lonergan, E.C. (1980, November). Humanizing the hospital experience: Report of a group program for needy patients. *Health and Social Work, 5*(4), 53-63.

Lonergan, E.C. (1982). *Group intervention: How to begin and maintain groups in medical and psychiatric settings*. New York: Aronson.

Lopez, D.J. & Getzel, G.S. (1984, September). Helping gay AIDS patients in crisis. *Social Casework, 65*(7), 387-94.

Lubell, D. (1986). Living with a lifeline: Peritoneal dialysis patients. In A. Gitterman & L. Shulman (Eds.), *Mutual aid groups and the life cycle* (pp. 283-295). Itasca, Ill.: F.E. Peacock.

Lurie, A., Rosenberg, G., & Pinsky, S. (Eds.). (1982). *Social work with groups in health settings*. New York: Prodist.

Mervis, P. (1983). Commentary. In G. Rosenberg & H. Rehr (Eds.), *Advancing social work practice in the health care field* (pp. 125-128). New York: The Haworth Press.

Northen, H. (1983). Social work groups in health settings: Promises and problems. In G. Rosenberg & H. Rehr (Eds.), *Advancing social work practice in the health care field* (pp. 107-121). New York: The Haworth Press.

Olson, M.M. (1986). When is it social work? Another look at practice with groups in health care. *Social Work in Health Care, 12*(1), 39-50.

Parad, H.J., Selby, L.G., & Quinlan, J. (1976). Crisis intervention in families and groups. In R.R. Roberts & H. Northen (Eds.), *Theories of social work groups* (pp. 304-330). New York: Columbia University Press.

Pueschel, S. & Yeatman, S. (1977, Fall). An emotional and counseling program for phenylketonuric adolescent girls and their parents. *Social Work in Health Care*, 3(1), 29-36.

Roback, H.B. (1984). Conclusion: Critical issues in groups approaches to disease management. In H.B. Roback (Ed.), *Helping patients and their families cope with medical problems* (pp. 527-543). San Francisco: Jossey-Bass.

Rosenberg, G. & Neill, G. (1982). Group services and medical illness: A review of the literature, 1964-1978. In A. Lurie, G. Rosenberg, & S. Pinsky (Eds.), *Social work with groups in health settings*. New York: Prodist.

Schopler, J.H. & Galinsky, M.J. (1985). The open-ended group. In M. Sundel, P. Glasser, R. Sarri, & R. Vinter (Eds.), *Individual change through small groups* (pp. 87-100). New York: Free Press.

Spink, D. (1976, November). Crisis intervention for parents of the deaf child. *Health and Social Work*, 1(4), 140-160.

Steinglass, P., Gonzalez, S., Dosovitz, L., & Reiss, D. (1982). Discussion groups for chronic hemodialysis patients and their families. *General Hospital Psychiatry*, 4(1), 7-14.

Strelnick, A.H. (1977). Multiple family group therapy: A review of the literature. *Family Process*, 16, 307-325.

Subramanian, K. (1986, Fall). Group training for the management of chronic pain in interpersonal situations. *Social Work with Groups*, 9(3), 55-69.

Subramanian, K. & Rose, S.D. (1985, Fall). Group treatment for the management of chronic pain. *Social Work Research and Abstracts*, 21, 29-30.

Weiner, H.J. (1959, October). The hospital the ward, and the patients as clients: Use of the group method. *Social Work*, 4(4).

White, P. & Baker, L. (1977, August). Group therapy with multiple sclerosis couples. *Health and Social Work*, 1(3), 188-195.

Whittaker, J.K. & Garbarino, J. (1983). *Social support networks: Informal helping in the social services*. New York: Aldine Publishing Co.

Yalom, I.D. (1970, 1975, 1985). *The theory and practice of group psychotherapy*. New York: Basic Books.

Young, C. (1957). Social group work with children in a general hospital. *Group work papers* (pp. 56-64). New York: National Conference of Social Work.

Developing a Group Program
in a Health Care Setting

M. Carlean Gilbert

SUMMARY. Social workers who create group programs in the health care setting must design programs that not only respond to the needs of the patients but also meet the needs of the organization. Social group workers' goals and interventions are identified as they relate to three major stages of program development: initiation, implementation, and stabilization. The advantages of the contingency model as an analytical framework are discussed, and illustrations from an open-ended support group for parents of hospitalized children are presented.

Group programs, not unlike other social work programs, purport to serve the best interests of the client. Political reality, however, mandates that successful group programs often must serve the best interests of the health care setting as well. In most situations clinical skills alone are insufficient to establish a viable group program. The social group worker also must possess the ability to analyze the organizational setting and to create an organizational structure that will support the program.

Neither success nor failure in developing a group program are random phenomena; there is a rich body of organizational theory to guide the practitioner's activities (Lorsch, 1977; Pfeffer & Salan-

M. Carlean Gilbert, ACSW, is affiliated with the Department of Social Work, The North Carolina Memorial Hospital, Chapel Hill, NC 27514.

The author appreciates the support of Ms. Jean Batten, ACSW, Ms. Barbara Wedehase, ACSW, co-leaders of the parents' group, and Ms. Juanita Todd, Chief of Pediatric Social Work, all of whom were colleagues at The North Carolina Memorial Hospital, Chapel Hill, NC. The author also wishes to thank Professor Mildred D. Mailick, City University of New York-Hunter College School of Social Work, for reviewing an earlier draft of this manuscript.

27

cik, 1977; Weick, 1977). Theory guides the social worker's design of a group program that can withstand the constant shifting of the fragmented, semi-autonomous systems that are characteristic of the health care setting. Analysis of the health care organization and design of the group program are enhanced by use of Glisson's contingency model for social welfare administration (Glisson, 1981). This paper presents some advantages and resistances to groupwork in the health care setting, describes the contingency model, and illustrates its application with examples from a parents' group at a university hospital.

ADVANTAGES AND RESISTANCES TO GROUPWORK IN HEALTH CARE SETTINGS

Groups in the health care setting can be effective, as indicated by an increasing number of publications describing their use since the mid-1960s (Carlton, 1986). Groups often can alleviate long-standing concerns about the accessibility, equity, and quality of health care services. Voluntary groups, especially, seem to be an appropriate fit with the consumer orientation of contemporary patients. The skyrocketing costs of medical care, the concomitant limitations on the worker's time and energy, and the increased demands for accountability from third-party guarantors necessitate cost-effective practice. Often one or two clinicians can meet the general needs of many patients through groups. Furthermore, groups increase exponentially the possible number of supportive relationships among members who share a common problem. Some patients respond better to a group approach rather than to an individual one because it offers opportunities for modeling, problem-solving, and indirect influences. Finally, clinicians benefit from stimulating alternatives to individual and family approaches, and this variation protects against the professional burnout that stems from repetition.

The social worker must also understand why there may be limited use of group programs in health care settings. A major reason for lack of support often is that the personnel and organizational structure tend to be strongly oriented toward the medical model with its emphasis on individual therapy, including psychosocial treatment (Gitterman, 1982). Some professionals maintain a bias toward long-term psychotherapy groups and thus fail to see the advantages of the open-ended or short-term support groups that are typical in a general hospital. In addition, some clinicians fear that they lack the expertise to do groupwork and prefer to function in safer, less visible individual relationships (Carlton, 1986; Sherman, 1979).

A CONCEPTUAL FRAMEWORK: THE CONTINGENCY MODEL

The contingency model for social welfare administration (Glisson, 1981) has several important advantages for analyzing the complex interrelationships of people within the health care setting. The basic premise of this model is that the determination of any appropriate action regarding program development is dependent upon the uniqueness of the organization and its current situation; there is no "best" program design. This comprehensive model serves as a useful framework because it: integrates aspects of general systems, human relations, and rational models of organizational theory; avoids prescribed approaches to program design; examines the special features of human service organizations; and recognizes that organizations experience developmental stages (Glisson, 1981). This model also is comfortable for clinicians because in many aspects it is analogous to individual, family, and group approaches.

The contingency model is a dynamic one that simultaneously considers six interrelated systems of the health organization: goals/values, structural, technological, psychosocial, environmental, and managerial. The following aspects of these subsystems affect the parents' group program:

1. The goals and values, admittedly a misnomer for a "subsystem," function as a boundary system because they direct policies, objectives, and constraints at all levels of the health care setting.
2. The structural subsystem describes the organizational structure, which is composed of varying degrees of job specialization, communications, hierarchy of authority, and reward systems.
3. The technological subsystem of organizations refers to the pre-

scribed sequence of worker activities, a process that often is indeterminate because of the unpredictability of the human beings.

4. The psychosocial subsystem describes aspects relevant to the social worker such as job satisfaction and compatibility with institutional values. These four subsystems, which are managed by administrators and embedded in a larger environmental system, compose the health care setting. Significantly, the contingency model does not assert that one subsystem is more important than another; however, it acknowledges that some subsystems exert more influence that others during certain stages of development or in particular institutions (Glisson, 1981). The social worker must continually evaluate the influences of these subsystems throughout all stages of program development.

Like effective clinical practice, program planning must be informed by theory rather than based on happenstance. The following discussion identifies and illustrates principles derived from the contingency model that enable the group worker to develop strategies for creating the essential "goodness of fit" between the group program and its organizational environment. Worker goals and interventions are presented as they relate to three major stages of program development: initiation, implementation, and stabilization (Patti, 1983; Weissman, 1983). Practice examples are drawn from an open-ended, voluntary support group for parents of hospitalized and chronically ill children. For nine years this social work group has met weekly or bi-weekly for one-hour sessions in a 620-bed teaching hospital. The group is generally composed of three to ten parents, the majority of whom are mothers; many parents have repeated attendance due to lengthy or multiple admissions of their children.

INITIATION STAGE

Essential factors to consider during the initiation stage include: identification of the need for a group program, acquisition of political and financial support, and creation of a program plan that will enhance current support and provide guidelines for later implementation. Social work groups may be initiated by organizational leaders who acquire new funding, desire to change the direction of an organization, or wish to try an innovation. Less frequently frontline workers seek change based on their direct experiences with patients (Patti, 1983, pp. 64-65).

> The specific planning instigator for the parents' group was the observation of several clinicians that parents met spontaneously in the ward lounge and thus demonstrated their need to share information, to gain support, and to socialize.

During the initiation phase a program is especially susceptible to political, economic, and administrative influences. There are two major goals during this vulnerable stage. First, the social worker must demonstrate through advance planning the capability to achieve the goals and objectives of authorized institutional policy. Second, the social worker must secure the necessary political and financial support from both internal and external constituencies in order for the program to gain legitimacy, to maintain its purpose, and to avoid alterations in its design. Political leverage points and coalitions must be analyzed in order to secure early and continual involvement of influential staff members (Patti, 1983, pp. 68-69). The key actors to be considered include: (a) providers of resources such as personnel, funding, raw materials, equipment, and physical space; (b) consumers; (c) competitors; and (d) regulatory groups (Thompson, 1967).

To acquire support, the social worker must possess or develop a power base. The major types of power generally accessible to the front-line worker are interpersonal and expert power. Interpersonal or referent power is the influence with others that is based upon interpersonal attraction and/or positive identification with the social work profession; expert power is based upon demonstration of professional knowledge and skills (Katz & Kahn, 1966, p. 344). Frequently, the worker's position within the organization determines the source, the amount, and the contingencies under which available power can be mobilized (Hasenfeld, 1974). One of the cheapest ways to acquire power is to build prestige (Thompson, 1967).

> A respected history of classroom and clinical teaching combined with media coverage of the parents' group and other social work projects enhanced the social workers' prestige in the hospital.

At this stage the actors in the internal environment such as chiefs of medical services and actors in the external environment such as legislative boards are likely to exert the most significant and long-lasting effects on program goals, values, and objectives (Glisson, 1981). In fact, they often determine the group's survival, especially when the social worker is dependent upon the organizational leaders of a host agency for information, support, and authorization (Patti, 1983, p. 65).

A careful analysis of the goals and values of the institution and its attendant subsystems is fundamental, for these constraints define the parameters of social work activities. The limitations that affect program development can be based upon tradition, religious affiliation, public policy, professional ideology, or funding patterns (Glisson, 1981). Most importantly, group goals must be compatible with institutional goals. Ineffective programs can result when the mission of the hospital or specialty service is vague or the group is initiated because of the personal interests of the professional rather than patient or institutional needs (Abramson, 1983).

> The three mandates of the illustrative hospital are clinical care, medical education, and research. Goals for the parents' group are consistent with quality clinical care because they are intended to strengthen adaptive behaviors of patients and their families and to prevent maladaptive ones. Specific group goals are clearly identified: to provide a safe accepting environment for verbalization of thoughts and feelings; to strengthen healthy coping mechanisms; to share information; and to offer socialization opportunities.

The decision to offer a group program must be based on the concept of unmet needs. Adequate assessment of patient and hospital needs is essential because: (a) it prevents premature closure on options; (b) it can be used by program advocates to gain political support and resources for the new group; (c) it provides baseline information that may be of later utility when the program is evaluated; and (d) it often determines where a program is located, especially if one assumes that there are always conflicting needs, limited resources, and variations in support. Being sensitive to possible competition from other professionals, the social worker may choose to create beneficial programs that focus on populations that are underserved due to another's lack of interest or expertise.

Unfortunately, the co-facilitators of the parents' group did not complete an initial needs assessment. This oversight led to disappointing attendance when paternalistic co-leaders assumed that the parents needed education on certain issues such as child development and announced pre-determined topics. Also, some parents expressed no need to attend the parents' group because they were already involved in community groups such as Association for Retarded Citizens or an existing hospital group for cancer patients.

Needs assessments are almost always constrained by limits of time, direct and indirect costs, professional expertise, and usefulness. In order to obtain the necessary support of the institution, the needs assessment must focus on staff perceptions of patient needs rather than on patient perceptions alone. It is important to contact all persons and existing programs that might interface with the group program in order to identify common concerns. The complexity of this task enlarges as the size of the institution increases; consensus, commonality of goals, and individual participation decrease with increased size whereas communication, control, and coordination difficulties increase.

In most health care settings the need for a high degree of predictability, coordination, and accountability results in a rigid hierarchy of authority, which has two lines. First, there is a hierarchical structure, which is based on varying levels of subordination; second, there is a lateral structure, which is defined by particular areas of expertise and function. It is politically wise for the social worker to identify whom to contact, what sequence of contacts to follow, and whether individual versus group meetings are appropriate.

These early contacts permit the social worker to understand other perspectives, to assess possible resistances, and to exchange information about what a group program is and importantly what it is not. For instance, a primary physician, who was trained to assume an authoritarian role in order to protect the patient during life and death crises, may feel that his or her control regarding patient welfare is threatened by a parent's involvement with other professionals.

A meeting with an influential physician who strongly objected to the proposed parents' group uncovered his strong fears that the meetings would become gripe sessions and would undermine his rapport and authority with parents. Empathizing with this concern, the social workers noted a recent ward incident in which a mother with borderline personality characteristics created considerable difficulty in parent-staff relationships by spreading false information. The group, they countered, would have been an ideal forum to clarify distortions and to decrease unwarranted parental anxieties. The physician gave his approval to the proposed program.

In another instance, a formal presentation to one medical department elicited differences between the professional norms of physicians and social workers. These physicians requested that a parent's attendance receive the physician's prior approval and that a parent's comments be documented in the medical report. Their professional stance conflicted with important social work values of confidentiality and freedom of choice, especially for the non-patient. An agreement was negotiated that relevant medical recording would be added to the child's medical record either with the parent's permission or in a potentially harmful situation.

During the needs assessment the worker can learn reasons for past successful and unsuccessful group programs, evaluate current problems from the viewpoints of the multi-disciplinary staff members, and identify factors that may enhance or impede establishment of the group program.

Facilitating optimal attendance, staff members provided practical information about admission and discharge patterns, daily scheduling of therapies, evaluations, academic tutoring, recreational activities, and even programming of children's television programs. The group met at 4 p.m., when children were entertained by "Sesame Street," on Wednesday, which had the highest hospital census. This time allowed parents to return to the rooms prior to evening medical rounds, and fathers who worked first shift could attend.

Timely and informative communication is essential throughout the initiation stage.

Following these informal contacts with hospital staff, the social workers sent memoranda describing the group, its goals, and its operational policies to all levels of hospital staff, e.g., hospital administrators, attending physicians, nurses, chaplains, other social workers, child psychologists, hospital school teachers, recreation therapists, physical therapists, volunteers, and ward secretaries. These memoranda were followed by additional correspondence, individual meetings with influential staff members, and formal presentations to some medical divisions. These activities enabled the social workers to discuss the group program with others and to adjust the program to fit with the health care system prior to implementation. Ultimately, social work supervisors, hospital administrators, and physicians sanctioned the proposal, the recreation therapy department provided playroom space, and the hospital volunteers funded the refreshments.

Successful completion of these initiation stage tasks can be a lengthy process of several months; the necessary chores can be mundane, time-consuming ones that may not be of intrinsic interest to the clinician. However, they are absolutely essential to successful program development.

IMPLEMENTATION STAGE

After the group program has been legitimized and resources have been obtained, implementation begins. During this stage the social group worker must accomplish two major programmatic goals. First, the program must establish a domain. Second, the program must develop environmental certainty with those organizations whose cooperation and resources are vital to its existence (Patti, 1983, pp. 112-113). Issues of domain, exchange, and equilibrium all impact upon the successfulness of the group program.

Prior to developing reciprocal relationships with members of the health care organization, the group program must acquire bargaining power by establishing domain. Domain defines the boundary points at which the program is dependent upon its environment for input, and it generally is identified by target populations, types of problems, and expertise. Traditionally, the domain of social work in health care settings has been a unique focus on the family of the patient, whose psychosocial needs must be met (Caroff & Mailick, 1985). Sometimes the establishment of a specific domain requires negotiations over diffuse functions or legitimization by other organizations (Levine & White, 1969). If a program monopolizes the provision of a resource needed in the health care setting, the program will have much power and autonomy (Thompson, 1967); conversely, if an unmet need is fulfilled by similar competitive programs or is non-essential, the power and autonomy of the program decrease.

On the pediatric services the norm, which is sanctioned formally by written protocols and informally by referral patterns, is that the family of the chronically ill child is the domain of the social worker. However, the hospital staff does not view the parents' group as a resource critical to the function of the pediatric service. Therefore, although the group program has clear domain in terms of boundaries and professional functions, the power and autonomy of the program are limited because the service is perceived as non-essential.

Simply stated, exchange occurs when two or more parties establish domain and trade resources in order to serve their own best interests. Homans introduced the concept of exchange to organizational theory, which suggests that individuals and groups are willing to pay a cost, e.g., money, personnel, referrals, in exchange for a reward (Homans, 1958). When the social worker is negotiating the terms of the exchange, he or she must resist the temptation to underbid services or to promise more than the group program can deliver. If commitments cannot be met, the program's credibility suffers; conversely, if excessive commitments are kept, they may be at the expense of over-extended staff and low morale (Patti, 1983, p. 125). The social worker also must remember that organizations exist in a pluralistic system. Each system exchanges with several other systems, and each of them has its own domain and organizational environment. The result is a complicated network of exchanges and interdependencies among patients, families, health care professionals, and support staff.

A rapid turnover in volunteers who are assigned to help with the parents' group by delivering and returning the refreshment cart existed. Discussion with the volunteers indicated that their "reward" for contributing services was interaction with hospitalized children. When we arranged for the volunteers to stay with very anxious children while their parents attended the group, volunteers were more likely to make a lengthy commitment to the program.

Issues related to changes in organizational equilibrium are also important to consider during implementation. The social worker is naive to assume that the group program will be welcomed automatically by others, for any new element upsets existing equilibrium and engenders resistance. Even when the program is well designed, there are unpredictable and unavoidable obstacles to implementation. Bardach (1977) describes these impediments to implementation in gamesmanship metaphors such as "tokenism," "massive resistance," and "piling on," which describe resistances of both providers and recipients to group programs.

"Tokenism" is a provider game in which providers of input resources appear to contribute but in reality make only a nominal or substandard contribution (Bardach, 1977, p. 98).

Pediatric social workers initially expressed eagerness to co-facilitate the parents' group, but their own service demands led first to postponements and later to firm decisions not to do the group. Thus, implementing and maintaining the group largely became the responsibility of those who initially had proposed it as a team project.

Physical space was generously donated by another department. However, its staff members had unanticipated needs to traffic the room, to make telephone calls, and to have staff conferences in adjacent offices during group sessions. These activities were distracting to both parents and co-leaders.

Although some impediments to a group program do not emerge until the implementation stage, the social worker can incorporate anti-tokenism strategies into the initial design. One anti-tokenism strategy is to "do without" a resource provided by others (Bardach, 1977, p. 103). Another strategy is for the social worker to provide the needed resource.

When the parents' group originally was proposed, colleagues enthusiastically agreed to urge parents to attend the group. However, their own professional commitments understandably took priority, and parents often were unaware of the program. Attendance was minimal, and clearly the group could not "do without" its most important input resource — parents. The co-leaders themselves assumed responsibility for recruiting parents by hanging posters and, most effectively, going to the patients' rooms and extending personal invitations. A marked increase in attendance resulted.

"Massive resistance," which is defined as large-scale non-compliance, is a second game that obstructs program implementation (Bardach, 1977, p. 108). It is played by recipients of a program who refuse to participate in it. One counter approach to "massive resistance" is the pseudo command, e.g., "come to the group," which is based on the assumption that most individuals are obedient (Bardach, 1977, pp. 110-12). Of course, the clinician must respect the rights of the parents to refuse services.

A common version of this game occurs when parents who are gathered in the waiting rooms decline the social worker's invitations to attend the parents' group and claim that they have their "own group right here." Sometimes an invitation is sufficient to encourage participation. When the parent might perceive himself or herself as a minority, such as the only father, the suggestion to bring a friend often results in two parents coming to the group. Another approach to encourage attendance is to use reinforcers. Sometimes a parent is attracted simply by the availability of refreshment. For another parent, the reinforcement is a place away from the child to safely ventilate sadness and fears regarding a devastating diagnosis.

Another impediment to implementation occurs when other professionals hang onto the coattails of a successful program and attempt to attach their own goals onto it, a game labeled "piling on" (Bardach, 1977, pp. 85-90). The collective effect of these enthusiastic responses not only may add to the group leaders' burdens but also can modify program goals.

Staff from social work, psychology, rehabilitation counseling, pastoral care, and nursing requested opportunities for their interns to observe or to co-lead the parents' group. These solicitations led to increased responsibilities for the social workers related to establishing eligibility criteria, orienting, supervising, and evaluating for allied-health students. These requests also necessitated re-negotiation with an influential physician, who had insisted that the group not be used for research or professional education, before interns participated.

Other impediments result from inanimate forces that simply wane over time. Problems of incompetence, variability, and insufficient coordination flow from this "social enthropy" (Bardach, 1977, pp. 125-139). Each of these problems were addressed during program implementation.

The first problem, incompetence, arises when the social workers responsible for an ongoing group program lack the clinical and/or organizational skills necessary to facilitate and to maintain it. Because it is particularly critical to demonstrate competence during the implementation stage, the recruitment, continuing education, and supervision of social group workers must become an institutionalized priority.

The parents' group program was aided by regular consultation with a professor of social group work. Such consultation provided continual support and stimulation, which were further increased by the participation of a social work intern.

A second problem occurs when variability among co-leaders, group compositions, and changing topics results in lack of continuity and standardization of practice. These inconsistencies tended to interfere with evaluation of the overall group program through content analyses, which was unreliable due to different styles of recording. Unexpectedly, however, the group recordings contributed to the continuity of the group.

Two co-leaders from a pool of three clinicians facilitate the group, which somewhat protects the group from negative impact of staff turnover. Since one of these two leaders also facilitates the next group, the legacy of the group is passed on. The passage and evolution of group norms, which also are transmitted through the recordings, are a major source of continuity and stabilization for the group.

A third problem is the coordination difficulty encountered when the social worker combines the activities of fragmented systems of the health care system. Poor coordination results in surpluses, shortages, and delays.

A seemingly minor arrangement for refreshments exemplifies the frustrating measures needed to correct coordination problems stemming from miscommunications, staff turnover, and logistics. Beverages and cookies were to be provided weekly by the hospital cafeteria service and funded by the hospital volunteers. Delivery of the refreshments varied from being prompt to late or non-existent; the order itself was either incomplete, duplicated, or substituted. The far-reaching steps necessary to create a standing food order required multiple telephone contacts and correspondence over several months among the social work department, food services, hospital volunteers, and ultimately the operations manager of the hospital.

In summary, the social workers' tasks during the implementation phase must be directed towards establishing a system of reciprocal relationships between the group program and other actors in the health care system. This goal requires demonstration of competence, definition of a functional domain, establishment of predictable exchange relationships, and an efficient and coordinated structure for the program within its organizational environment.

STABILIZATION STAGE

Stabilization or institutionalization of the group program represents completion of initiation and implementation tasks and commencement of others. Although many aspects of the implementation phase overlap with the stabilization phase, the emphasis shifts to maintenance of a quality program, which has become a permanent part of the health care system.

Three goals must be achieved: (a) creating an environment that promotes high level performance of the group leaders; (b) establishing a method for program evaluation; and, (c) structuring the program to cope with internal and external environmental changes (Patti, 1983, p. 162).

Creation of an environment that fosters competent group leaders includes ongoing commitment of the social work department. This commitment is reflected in formal policy statements and operational goals that are directed at sustaining quality recruitment and staff development, examples of which are listed in the previous section. Rewards such as merit raises, promotions, benefits, release time, involvement in professional organizations, special titles, and public recognition as well as the intrinsic rewards of increased skills and knowledge can be used to induce clinicians to participate in the group program.

Evaluation becomes a basis for monitoring the effectiveness of the group program, modifying it when needed, guiding decision-making, and providing feedback to political and financial supporters.

Several methods for evaluating the group program are utilized. Content analyses are made of now-standardized group recordings, which include dates, members present, seating arrangements, common themes, interventive strategies, children's diagnoses, and clinician's impressions of the session. The most frequent topics generated by parents include utilizing hospital services, dealing with separation anxiety, and developing adaptive coping mechanisms. Identification of these recurrent themes results in improved program planning, professional education, and clinical preparation by the group leaders. These evaluations also are a source of feedback to physicians, whose initial concerns about gripe sessions have been allayed.

Survey instruments are distributed periodically to parents in order to evaluate their unmet needs, obstacles to attendance, and reactions to participation in the group.

Lastly, the group program must be structured to withstand both internal and external environmental changes. To withstand internal programmatic changes, the group must receive a staffing commitment from the social work department.

One source of difficulty flows from the continual loss of committed, experienced, and skilled group leaders due to staff turnover. The program eventually became a service of the pediatric social work team rather than only the program innovators, which broadened the base of support for the group program.

To withstand external influences, financial and spatial resources are legitimized by hospital administration and confirmed in writing. Periodic memoranda and personal contacts provide communication to health care professionals whose ongoing support is needed and information to new staff members who may be unaware of the group program.

During the stabilization stage of development there may be no plans for expansion of the program. In fact, the parents' group described throughout this discussion has existed nine years with minor adjustments to its changing environment. However, the goals of structuring a program that adjusts to internal and external environmental changes, promotes high level performance of clinical staff, and is regularly evaluated continue to be necessary for maintenance of a quality group program.

CONCLUSION

The social workers who develop a group program in a health care setting must create a program that fits the needs of the organization as well as responds to the needs of the patient. The contingency model provides a framework for identifying the goals and interventions needed to secure the necessary internal and external support for the program during its unique phases of initiation, implementation, and stabilization. Contrary to some popular thought, focus on the institutional needs enhances rather than detracts from group service to patients. As Abramson writes, "The client-centered focus is a necessary but not sufficient basis for program development" (Abramson, 1983, p. 186). The successful social group worker must be not only a skilled clinician but also a politically and organizationally astute program developer.

REFERENCES

Abramson, J. (1983). A non-client-centered approach to program development in a medical setting. In H. Weissman, I. Epstein, & A. Savage (Eds.), *Agency-based social work*, (pp. 178-186). Philadelphia: Temple University Press.

Bardach, E. (1977). *The implementation game*. Cambridge, MA: MIT Press.

Carlton, T. O. (1986). Group process and group work in health social work practice. *Social Work with Groups*, *9*(2), 5-20.

Caroff, P. & Mailick, M. (1985). The patient has a family: reaffirming social work's domain. *Social Work in Health Care*, *10*(4), 17-34.

Galinsky, M. J. & Schopler, J. H. (1974). The social work group. In J. B. Shaffer & M. D. Galinsky, *Models of group therapy and sensitivity training*, (pp. 19-48). Englewood Cliffs, NJ: Prentice-Hall.

Galinsky, M. J. & Schopler, J. H. (1985, Summer). Patterns of entry and exit in open-ended groups. *Social Work with Groups*, *8*(2), 67-80.

Garvin, C. D. & Glasser, P. H. (1974). The bases of social treatment. In P.

Glasser, R. Sarri, & R. Vinter (Eds.), *Individual change through small groups*, (pp. 483-507). New York: The Free Press.

Germain, C. B. (1984). *Social work practice in health care*. New York: The Free Press.

Germain, C. B. & Gitterman, A. (1980). *The life model of social work practice*, (pp. 343-365). New York: Columbia University Press.

Gitterman, A. (1982). The use of groups in health settings. In A. Lurie, G. Rosenberg, & S. Pinsky (Eds.), *Social work with groups in health settings*, (pp. 6-24). New York: Prodist.

Glisson, C. A. (1981). A contingency model of social welfare administration. *Administration in Social Work*, 5(1), 15-29.

Hasenfeld, Y. (1974). Organizational factors in services to groups. In P. Glasser, R. Sarri, & R. Vinter (Eds), *Individual change through small groups*, (pp. 307-322). New York: The Free Press.

Homans, G. C. (1969). The Western Electric Researches. In A. Etzioni (Ed.), *Readings on modern organizations*, (pp. 99-114). Englewood Cliffs: Prentice-Hall.

Katz, D. & Kahn, R. (1966). Leadership. In *The social psychology of organizations*, (pp. 300-335). New York: John Wiley.

Levine, S. & White, P. (1969). Exchange as conceptual framework for the study of interorganizational relationships. In A. Etizioni (Ed.), *A sociological reader on complex organizations*, (pp. 117-132). New York: Holt, Reinhart, & Winston.

Lindamood, M. M. & Klein, E. (1983). In L. Hubschman (Ed.), *Hospital social work practice*, (pp. 105-116). USA: Praeger.

Lorsch, J. W. (1977). Organizational design: a situational perspective. *Organizational Dynamics*, 6, 16-29.

Patti, R. J. (1983). *Social welfare administration: managing social problems in a developmental context*. Englewood Cliffs: Prentice-Hall.

Pfeffer, J. & Salancik, G. (1977). Organizational design: the case for a coalitional model of organizations. *Organizational Dynamics*, 6, 15-29.

Shaffer, J. B. & Galinsky, M. D. (1974). *Models of group therapy and sensitivity training*. Englewood Cliffs: Prentice-Hall.

Sherman, E. (June, 1979). *Social work with groups in a hospital setting*. Paper presented at a conference on "Social Work with Groups in Maternal and Child Health," New York.

Thompson, J. D. (1967). *Organizations in action: social science bases of administrative theory*, (pp. 25-38). New York: McGraw Hill.

Weick, K. E. (1977). Organization design: organizations as self-designing systems. *Organizational Dynamics*, 6, 31-46.

Weissman, H., Epstein, I., & Savage, A. (1983). *Agency-based social work*, (pp. 169-200). Philadelphia: Temple University Press.

Making Teams Work

Julie S. Abramson

SUMMARY. Social workers are important participants in teams in health and mental health settings, functioning as members, leaders and consultants. Therefore, the development of effective teamwork skills is critical for social workers. This article articulates those skills, strategies and attitudes that enhance team functioning. Approaches generic to all roles are presented, and then those specific to a team member, leader or consultant are outlined.

Although group process factors affecting teamwork have been identified in the literature (Ducanis & Golin, 1979; Kane, 1975), there has been little exploration of appropriate interventions to influence team process. As active team participants in health and mental health settings, social workers have many opportunities to contribute to effective team functioning. This article will articulate some of the skills, strategies and attitudes that social workers can use as team leader, member or consultant. Before proceeding, however, it is important to examine obstacles to effective teamwork so that strategies are developed with these in mind.

OBSTACLES TO EFFECTIVE TEAMWORK

The interdisciplinary health care team is widely viewed as the primary vehicle for providing comprehensive, coordinated care to clients. In fact, both Kane (1975) and Halstead (1976) agree that the team is so accepted as a mechanism of service delivery that other

Julie S. Abramson, PhD, is Assistant Professor at the School of Social Welfare, State University of New York at Albany, 135 Western Avenue, Albany, NY 12222.

The author gratefully acknowledges the comments of Ronald Toseland.

45

alternatives are rarely considered. Nevertheless, much of the literature on teams examines perceived obstacles to effective team functioning.

Teams by definition bring together practitioners from different
professions with the expectation of developing consensus on approaches to patient care. Yet each profession socializes its members
differently in relation to which values, definitions of professional
role and models of intervention are imparted. Language, customs
and general professional culture can be so distinctive to each profession as to obscure common ground (Huntington, 1981). For instance, most social workers working with house staff physicians
can recall their shock at hearing physicians in training disparage
categories of patients as "crocks" or "turkeys" or using other pe-
jorative labels. Fox (1980) explains such behavior as an outlet for
expressing frustration with the uncertainties of medicine. Mizrahi
(1986) sees it as a reaction to the contrast between housestaff expectations of the training process and the realities of patient care.

Social workers, schooled in being non-judgmental, have little
tolerance for such physician responses. Physicians, on the other
hand, often identify social workers as "bleeding hearts" who will
help even the "undeserving." The vast gap between these two professional world views is but one example of the impact of differen-
tial socialization on collaborative relationships (Gartner, 1975).
Similar differences can be found between other professions as
well (Campbell-Heider & Pollack, 1987; Fessler & Adams, 1985;
Hulme, Bach & Lewis, 1988; Kulys & Davis, 1987) but are rarely
recognized as the cause of communication difficulties on teams
(Buckholdt & Gubrium, 1979).

Teams which include physicians often confront the continuing
dominance of physicians over medical and team decision making
(Abramson & Mizrahi, 1987; Dingwall, 1982; Freidson, 1970;
Nagi, 1975; New, 1968; Watt, 1985). In fact, physicians are less
likely to be team members than are other professionals (Kane,
1980; Toseland et al., 1986). Rotation of physicians through a unit
often necessitates continual team reconstitution (Lowe & Herranen,
1981). However, when present, they are almost always defined as
team leaders (Campbell-Heider & Pollock, 1987; Lowe & Herranen, 1981; Nagi, 1975). Their higher status disproportionately

influences team interaction, decision making, problem definition and options for intervention (Chapman, 1986; Ducanis & Golin, 1979; Toseland et al., 1986). In addition, physicians continue to be primarily male (although percentages are decreasing), while team members from most other professions are primarily women. Therefore, team interactions are influenced by traditional patterns of male dominance in social relationships (Lonergan, 1985; Huntington, 1981; Kerson, 1980).

Medical training with its emphasis on self-reliance and autonomy (Bucher & Stelling, 1977; Mizrahi & Abramson, 1985) inadequately prepares physicians for roles as either team leader or team member. Boerma (1987) suggests a need for reorientation training that would emphasize team functioning but also notes, as do others, that physicians are usually less motivated to participate in teamwork than other health care professionals (Mizrahi & Abramson, 1985; Nagi, 1975; Weissman, Epstein & Savage, 1983). In addition, frequently professed team norms of equality cause feelings of dissonance in team members when they confront the everyday reality of medical dominance (New, 1968).

Role competition is one of the most frequently discussed obstacles to effective teamwork. The priority given to professional allegiances by team members can lead to confrontations over "turf" as can problems with role clarity or role overlap (Kane, 1975; Lowe & Herranen, 1978; Watt, 1985). Interprofessional competition is also reinforced by dual lines of accountability for each team member (Banta & Fox, 1972). Responsibility for supervision, performance evaluation, promotion and continuing professional education are usually formally located within each profession rather than within the team. This may reduce motivation for team participation and diminish the significance of team decision making.

Despite the potential for conflict, teams usually operate under the premise that they can reach consensus on assigned tasks. This task focus can limit efforts to deal with the process issues related to overall team functioning, particularly conflict (Buckholdt & Gubrium, 1979; Ducanis & Golin, 1979). Furthermore, identification with the team and the desire for consensus and positive interprofessional relationships can lead members to minimize differences. Such pressures toward conformity can reduce consideration of alternatives or limit the freedom of team members to advocate for client interests if a challenge to other team members is involved (Abramson, 1984; Connaway, 1975; Mailick & Ashley, 1982).

Finally, teamwork takes place within an organizational context where factors external to the team may seriously influence options and resources available to the team (Watt, 1985; Lowe & Herranen, 1981; Nagi, 1975). For example, if the directors of social work and nursing are competing for control of a proposed home care program, team members from each discipline may act out some of the tensions between their administrators. At times team members might be transferred, based on budgetary problems or reallocation of priorities in an organization. In other situations, team treatment models might become less appropriate if modifications in organizational admission policies bring about changes in the client population served.

SKILLS FOR ENHANCING TEAM FUNCTIONING

Given the significant impact of the issues described above, it is remarkable that so many teams do function effectively. Social work team participants, drawing on clinical skills and experience can assist teams in a variety of ways. Dana (1983, p. 190) points out the relevance for team work of the "time-honored attributes of social work behavior" including: (a) beginning where one's colleagues are; (b) respect for differences in values, knowledge, and problem-solving styles; (c) willingness to share one's own knowledge, values and skills even when they may conflict with those held by others; (d) capacity   to work through rather than to avoid conflict; and (e) openness to the ideas and insights of others.

GENERIC SKILLS FOR TEAMWORK

Many of the most useful skills that social workers can employ in teamwork are drawn from work with groups. These include assessing the team as a group, contracting, monitoring of the process, dealing with conflict and understanding interprofessional differences.

Social workers who wish to contribute to effective team functioning must operate from the premise that the team is a group and that group process issues are affecting the capacity of the team to deliver services to patients (Kane, 1975). As obvious as this notion seems, it easily gets overlooked by a group of professionals focused on delivering patient care. Yet as Shulman (1982, p. 221) notes, so often "attention to the process leads directly to work on the task."

Lack of a clear contract is the source of many difficulties for both task and treatment groups. Contracting is a major problem in teams because the contract is usually presumed and rarely explicitly dealt with (Shulman, 1982). When a team is first being developed or is at a point of restructuring, all participants need a clear understanding of how the team will operate in relation to attendance, participation, composition, leadership, decision making, allocation of responsibilities and treatment models (Kahn, 1974). So often, these critical factors in team functioning get structured by default or tradition. Frequently, the leader simply establishes a particular mode of operation and the other team members follow suit. Efforts at recontracting can be generated by members, leaders or an outside consultant. The group can focus on clarifying or modifying the overall team purpose and structure. At times, intervention may be required to clarify the contract for a particular session.

It is also critical that one or more team participants maintain an overview of the team process, both within a given team meeting and from session to session. Such monitoring requires the ability to think simultaneously about treatment and team issues, and comfort in shifting back and forth in focus. This perspective allows the individual to assess team dynamics at a given point, to identify the issues underlying an atmosphere of tension or unproductivity, and then to develop a strategy to address the problem. Support can also be provided to others who take initiative for working on group process issues. The following vignette illustrates such an intervention.

At a team meeting in a rehabilitation hospital, the team leader, who was a physician, mentioned that he would begin interviewing applicants for the position of team psychologist. The former psychologist had been involved in some jurisdictional conflicts with the consulting psychiatrist, the nurse clinician and the social workers. The team leader did not seem to expect any discussion of his announcement and proceeded to review the patient roster for the week. Each team member presented a case for which the intake assessment had been completed. However, the usual exchanges about appropriate treatment approaches did not take place. The leader seemed baffled, asked for people's opinions several times, and then just made the decisions himself.

Finally, one of the occupational therapists commented that everyone sure was quiet today. That remark created more silence. Then one of the social workers said that she didn't know if other people were also preoccupied, but she knew that her mind was on the possibility of a new psychologist and whether the same problems would exist with a new person. When several heads nodded affirmatively, she wondered if it would be helpful, either in the meeting now or possibly as a subgroup later, to discuss the job description for this person. The team leader said he knew there had been some problems, but maybe he wasn't as aware of them as they were. Several people volunteered to meet with him after the meeting to discuss it further.

Skills in dealing with conflict and in consensus building are also essential for those team participants who wish to assist team development. The evolution of true consensus and growth in team functioning often depends on the ability of group members to confront conflict within the group directly (Northen, 1988; Whitaker, 1975; Zastrow, 1989). It may be necessary to discuss usually taboo areas if substantive agreement about key aspects of team process or patient care is to be achieved.

Often, safer issues can be tackled initially so that a reservoir of positive experiences in dealing with conflict can be used to create a new group culture (Deutsch, 1973). For example, during initial stages of team development, most mental health teams could safely discuss differing perspectives on treatment in a particular case. If however, the most powerful team member promotes a particular treatment model that is not well accepted by other team members, the challenge to authority implicit in discussing other approaches

would be much more threatening. It is best to confront such underlying conflicts after prior successes in resolving manifest problems.

Toseland and Rivas (1984) note a number of strategies that can
help a task group come to a resolution of differences. These include: (a) helping members to recognize the conflict and to express
the reasoning behind conflicting opinions and alternatives; (b) utilizing decision criteria jointly agreed on; (c) identifying the acceptable and unacceptable aspects of each alternative; and (d) subse-
quently combining the acceptable parts of several alternatives into
one solution. Broader conflicts can be divided into component parts
(Gouran, 1982) and consensus gained incrementally while clarifying misperceptions and distortions (Deutsch, 1973). Moreover,
modeling a professional demeanor, even in the fact of deeply felt
differences, maintains a "politeness ritual" which effectively
evokes and activates norms of responsibility in dealing with others
(Mikula & Schwinger, 1978).

Resolving conflict inevitably involves some redistribution of
power. Therefore, to facilitate resolution, it is critical to structure the
bargaining process to avoid a total win or lose situation (Deutsch,
1973; Gouran, 1982). Reframing a contending perspective in terms
of others' needs or ideology can assist the search for common
ground. For example, a social worker interested in obtaining service for a client might stress the potential for learning from a specific case when presenting it at an intake meeting in a training setting.

If, however, dissension is not overtly expressed, other approaches are needed. It is crucial to be alert to indications of conflict such as exchanges of glances among members, loss of eye
contact, evidence of irritation or frustration, subgroup talking, sar-
castic or sub rosa remarks and even physical restlessness. Such behavior should stimulate other participants to seek out the underlying
meaning. Inquiry and exploration are also necessary where disagreement is verbal, although indirectly expressed. Support should
be provided to a team member whose effort to raise an issue has
been avoided, cut off, ignored or diverted by the team leader or a
subgroup. When the issues are interpersonal, a direct approach
within the team meeting is often anxiety provoking and should only
be selected when the conflict between individuals is clearly interfer-

ing with the work of the team, i.e., it has in fact become a group problem.

Whichever type of conflict is influencing the team process, consensus is most likely to develop through the frequent reiteration and reinforcement of unifying themes. It is important to note however that consensus does not necessarily represent unanimous agreement but rather implies that all members can go along with the prevailing point of view and carry it out where necessary (Napier & Gershenfeld, 1981).

Finally, team participants need to understand the varying socialization experiences of each profession in relation to values, role of the provider, perspectives on patient care, and attitudes and preparation for teamwork (Compton & Galaway, 1984; Mizrahi & Abramson, 1985). When such understanding exists, behavior formerly attributed to individual personality factors becomes comprehensible as a product of professional socialization and therefore less personally alienating. Acknowledgement of the patterned responses of various professionals makes it possible to develop strategies to influence team processes that take these differences into account. For example, awareness of the norm of self reliance among housestaff physicians will help social workers and nurses to take the initiative if they want to be influential in patient management (Huntington, 1981).

SKILLS SPECIFIC TO ROLES AS TEAM LEADER, MEMBER OR CONSULTANT

The generic skills articulated above enhance the group process aspects of team functioning and can be utilized by social workers in any relationship to a team. However, some skills are more particular to the roles of leader, member or consultant. Interventions appropriate to each of these roles will now be discussed.

Skills as a Team Leader

Social workers serve as team leaders in many settings, although more often perhaps, in psychiatric than medical units. It is less likely that social workers will be the designated team leaders where physicians are also on the team, unless the unit or program has been developed by non physician staff or the physician is only present for case consultation. The norm of equality among participants promoted in many mental health programs can lead to rotating leadership or to assignment of the role to the best qualified person. In such programs, social workers are often team leaders. However, the tendency for physicians to dominate decision making even where others are designated as leaders may be a factor that social work team leaders will need to address. This can best be done by maintaining active leadership while acknowledging and supporting physician contributions.

There are many skills that a team leader can utilize to make teams function more effectively. Some skills such as conflict resolution and consensus building and the ability to keep an overview of the group process have been enumerated. Others include: (a) creating an atmosphere in the team that is conducive to problem solving; (b) identifying obstacles to problem solving; and (c) developing an administrative structure for the team.

The leader usually has major responsibility for creating an atmosphere and culture for group functioning and problem solving. Modeling or encouraging the open and rational discussion of differences can assist in the developing of a culture that helps teams to confront underlying conflicts successfully. In addition, the leader needs to communicate an optimistic view of the potential for change and of the capacities of the members to resolve the problems at hand. The leader thus provides support while simultaneously requesting the team to engage in problem solving.

The leader can mediate differences in professional status of team members by offering support to those who wish to raise differences with higher status team members or by simply promoting active participation by lower status team members. Sometimes the leader can utilize the safety of his/her position to question a generally accepted assumption or mode of operating. For example, the leader may choose to challenge assumptions about which team members see which type of patients. This pattern can be questioned directly or, using a particular patient as a point of departure, the discussion can be directed toward an evaluation of who has the best relationship, skills or experience to work most successfully with the client. Thus, tradition is eroded and new perspectives are introduced.

A good team leader tries to create a sense of identification with the whole team, despite the pull of various intraprofessional commitments, ideologies and loyalties (Watt, 1985). This can only succeed if the leader does not over-identify with his/her own profession and is perceived as even-handed in territorial disputes (Sheidel & Crowell, 1979). If possible, a culture eliminating professional jargon should be promoted. The leader also helps the team differentiate the resolvable conflicts from those which are intrinsic to life on a particular team.

Certain administrative activities facilitate team functioning. These include arranging for an appropriate physical setting, scheduling, preparing agendas and developing mechanisms for identifying those clients in need of review. Orientation of new members should be a formal process (Hooyman, 1984). Efforts to clarify or restate the team contract also need to be made at regular intervals (Shulman, 1982), stimulated by difficulties in team processes or by a significant amount of staff turnover.

Team leaders need to prepare for team meetings by "tuning in" (Shulman, 1984) to those team concerns likely to stir up feelings. In anticipating these, the leader assesses the current status of team relationships as preparation for developing relevant interventions during the team meeting (Scheidel & Crowell, 1979).

Many of the leader's responsibilities are more subtly defined. An effective leader can help team members avoid burnout and provide better care by recognizing when the team has developed norms that may be having a negative impact on patients (Joffee, 1979; Weissman, Epstein & Savage, 1983). Frequently, teams and team members lose the capacity to individualize certain categories of clients, particularly those with a poor prognosis (Maslach, 1978) or for whom available interventions do not easily succeed. An alert leader needs to identify such patterns and call the members' attention to them. Opportunities to reflect on these issues, away from the routines of patient care through a retreat, can assist staff to develop other strategies. In such situations, the team leader functions almost as a participant observer, analyzing the meaning of communication about patients and about the way they are categorized and treated

(Buckholdt & Gubrium, 1979). This role requires an ability to disengage oneself somewhat from "the way things are" in order to gain a renewed vision. The following example illustrates such a situation.

> Team members in an out-patient clinic for substance abusers had begun to set very limited treatment objectives for low income clients. The team leader assessed this response as relating to a disproportionate number of treatment failures with this group of clients. She observed team members gradually withdrawing from this population and decided to raise the issue at a team meeting. After evoking much frustrated commentary from the team members, she suggested that there might be other approaches that the team could develop to work more successfully with such clients. She proposed a workshop that would have components of specialized training with a consultant, followed by brainstorming sessions to integrate the consultant's input with the extensive knowledge already available within the team.

Finally, an effective team leader may need to work on some team problems outside the team meeting, through discussions with individual team members (Shulman, 1982). This might be done to provide support or feedback to a team member about his/her impact on the team process. In some situations, the leader might form a subcommittee of the team to bring suggestions for resolution of a particular problem to the team for discussion.

Skills as a Team Member

Team members are also a source of leadership on teams despite the absence of a formally designated role. In fact, where the formal leader lacks good team building skills, members may need to take greater initiative to facilitate team process. Bertcher (1987) points out that team members can offer leadership without undercutting the formal team leader. However, members must anticipate the leader's reaction to an intervention and insure that it will not be perceived as a competitive bid for leadership. Members can enhance team functioning through utilizing self assessment and assessment of team process, by providing support for others and through idea generation.

Any team member can provide the team with an assessment of team dynamics or can request that the team work on an identified issue. For example, a social work member of a dialysis team may feel that a team decision to transfer a patient to another dialysis center is the result of staff difficulties in dealing with this patient's admittedly difficult personality rather than based on medical needs. As a team member, she might raise this with the rest of the team by reflecting on her own mixed feelings toward this patient. Depending on the response to her openness, she could state her concern that feelings about this patient could easily contaminate the planning process. While functioning as a patient advocate, she also is contributing to norm development in relation to self awareness.

Support for others who risk entry into a taboo area can be critical at times. Ephross and Vassil (1987) suggest that supporting or building on another team member's idea encourages team cohesiveness and bonding as well as assisting in the development of a climate of mutual aid. Initiative can also be taken outside of team meetings to build support for tackling sensitive problems (Bernstein, 1973). For instance, a team member might arrange for several colleagues to illustrate a point she plans to bring up in a team meeting.

Team members can influence team process by freely expressing new ideas, even those not yet fully formed, in order to stimulate the thinking of others. Scheidel and Crowell (1979, p. 60) note however, that any contribution should be "in tune with the group goal." Encouraging the participation of quieter team members can enrich problem solving as can translating a useful comment that has been poorly stated or gone unnoticed (Bertcher, 1987; Hooyman, 1984). Attitudes toward ideas of other members can also facilitate or inhibit effective teamwork. The evaluation of another's ideas needs to be done without regard for the status or personal appeal of the individual or for his/her subgroup affiliations (Fisher & Ury, 1983). If such behavior is modeled by a team member, it can evoke similar responses from others. It is also important to contain feelings of anxiety and fear when changes are proposed and to remain open to new ideas (Scheidel & Crowell, 1979). When proposing change or confronting anxiety provoking issues, ideas should be framed in a way that permits others to redefine them or even deny them.

Individuals will have particular personal strengths and weaknesses as team members. Some will be more effective at facilitating the socioemotional aspects of the team process while others will be better able to help the team with tasks (Bales & Slater, 1955). Awareness of one's assets and vulnerabilities as a team member is crucial in selecting the most appropriate areas for intervention in the team process. Each member needs to monitor the impact of his/her personality on the group through awareness of personal verbal, non verbal and affective communication styles. Burghardt (1982, p. 29) urges individuals to confront the "personal realities of tactical implementation."

Skills as a Consultant to Teams

Social workers with particular areas of expertise have often provided consultative services to individual social workers and to social work programs (Shulman, 1987). In interdisciplinary settings, social workers have functioned as consultants to assist other groups of professionals such as nurses, physicians, medical students, psychiatric residents or teachers to learn relevant psychosocial content and techniques to facilitate interviewing or work with families (Kadushin, 1977). The potential clearly exists for social workers to function as consultants to teams in a variety of settings, although information is lacking about the frequency with which they fulfill this role.

Many social work skills, as noted earlier, are easily adapted to the milieu of the team (Rosenberg & Nitzberg, 1980). Those specific to the consultative role would include (1) problem assessment; (2) problem definition; (3) mediation and negotiation; and (4) contract development. The stated goal or agenda of the consultation is to bring about some change, either within the process, the structure or knowledge base of the team (Spencer & Croley, 1963).

Issues of trust, access, sponsorship and power need to be addressed if the outside consultant is to gather accurate information about problems and effectively engage the team members in problem solving efforts. The consultant must establish credibility and expertise, particularly with team members of higher status such as physicians. This can be assisted by having the team member who initiates the consultation share the consultant's resume, relevant publications and past history of successful consultative efforts with the rest of the team. Preliminary contacts with key individuals can also facilitate the development of confidence in the consultant.

Special status as outside expert does provide a unique source of leverage to the consultant, making it possible to focus on typically taboo areas such as inadequate leadership, interpersonal problems, or status concerns. For example, in one situation, the consultant helped the physician and non physician staff discuss the presumption that the physician's time was more valuable than that of others.

Effective consultation has been defined as involving a number of phases (Watkins, Holland & Ritvo, 1976). The first phase involves evaluation of motivation followed by data collection and assessment. A proposal for intervention is made and carried out and finally, feedback is provided.

Initially, the consultant needs to explore the reasons for having consultation at this point. The various expectations of the different team members and leaders need to be identified. An assessment needs to be made of the degree of support for the consultative process from different segments of the team. The information gathered in the first phase is then evaluated to identify patterns and areas of common concern as well as those specific to certain subgroups.

The structure of the consultative sessions needs to vary with service responsibilities, the goals of the consultation and with the problems uncovered during the assessment phase. Weekly one hour sessions with rotating attendance were the best solution for a group of emergency room staff concerned about staff interactions with relatives of patients. An outpatient clinic team was able to have a more concentrated opportunity to work on team problems at an all day retreat.

Specific approaches also should be tailored to particular characteristics of the team. With the emergency room staff group, scripts of common interactions between staff and relatives of patients were developed that illustrated typical exchanges. The staff were asked to role play these by re-writing the scripts to illustrate more successful ways of dealing with patients' relatives. The choice to work this way rather than to use open-ended role plays was made to lessen the degree of risk and exposure for team members in a group where no norm of sharing had been established previously.

With the clinic team, the choice was made to speak initially with the physician and non physician groups separately, based on the different degree of power residing in the two subgroups. In each subgroup, members were encouraged to raise issues related to those in the other subgroup at a later joint meeting. There was an effort to get commitment from one or more individuals to do so. When the total team convened, some didactic material was presented on professional socialization, both in general and specifically relating to the physician. This was done to set the stage for looking at some of the interprofessional issues and also as a safer, less personal way to enter discussion of differences among team members. The full team sessions then discussed some of the issues already identified such as different attitudes between the physicians and non physicians about the importance of research, and the need for a recommitment to a scheduled team meeting time.

The final phase should involve efforts to clarify what the consultation has accomplished and the development of next steps. A timetable should be established with responsibility for follow through delegated to specific individuals. In some situations, a plan is made for a follow up session. A final report should be issued by the consultant which summarizes the problems identified and solutions proposed.

The consultant has certain advantages in working with the team process that are not available to those in other roles. The authority mantle of the outside expert allows for greater latitude and risk taking in intervention. Also, the consultant, as outsider, is less concerned about his/her status in the group. As a result, there is greater freedom to be directive, to challenge traditional patterns and generally to be somewhat more confrontational than in the other roles. It can be helpful for the consultant to raise those issues identified as most threatening, in order to protect anxious team members. However, some of the preparatory work discussed above will insure that team members will then pick up on the openings provided by the consultant.

CONCLUSION

Social work practice skills, particularly those drawn from group work, are easily adapted to working with teams as a member, leader or consultant. As frequent participants in teams, social workers are in an excellent position to apply the strategies and skills outlined here. Opportunities to function as team leaders and consultants are increasing as the contributions of social workers to facilitating both the process and tasks of teams are recognized.

REFERENCES

Abramson, J. & Mizrahi, T. (1986). Strategies for enhancing collaboration between social workers and physicians. *Social Work in Health Care, 12*(1), 1-21.

Abramson, M. (1984). Collective responsibility in interdisciplinary collaboration: An ethical perspective for social workers. *Social Work in Health Care, 10*(1), 35-43.

Bales, R. & Slater, P. (1955). Role differentiation in small decision making groups. In T. Parsons & R. Bales (Eds.), *Family, socialization and interaction process*. New York: Free Press.

Banta, H.D. & Fox, R. (1972). Role strains of a health care team in a poverty community. *Social Science and Medicine, 6*, 697-722.

Bernstein, S. (1973). Conflict and group work. In S. Bernstein (Ed.), *Explorations in group work* (pp. 72-106). Boston: Charles River Books.

Bertcher, H. (1987). Effective group membership. *Social Work with Groups, 10*(2), 57-67.

Boerma, T. (1987). The concept of a primary health care team in developing countries. *Social Science and Medicine, 25*(6), 747-752.

Bucher, R. & Stelling, J. *Becoming professional*. Beverly Hills: Sage Publications.

Buckholdt, D. & Gubrium, J. (1979). Doing staffings. *Human Organization, 38*(3), 255-264.

Burghardt, S. (1982). *Organizing for community action*. Beverly Hills: Sage Publications.

Campbell-Heider, N. & Pollack, D. (1987). Barriers to physician/nurse collegiality: An anthropological perspective. *Social Science and Medicine, 25*(5), 421-425.

Compton, B. & Galaway, B. (1984). *Social work processes* (3rd ed.). Homewood, IL: The Dorsey Press.

Connaway, R. (1975). Teamwork and social worker advocacy: Conflicts and possibilities: *Community Mental Health Journal, 11*(4), 381-388.

Dana, B. (1983). The collaborative process. In R. Miller & H. Rehr (Eds.),

Social work issues in health care (pp. 181-220). Englewood Cliffs, NJ: Prentice-Hall.

Deutsch, M. (1973). *The resolution of conflict*. New Haven: Yale University Press.

Dingwall, R. (1982). Problems of team work in primary care. In A. Clare & R. Carney (Eds.), *Social work and primary care* (pp. 81-103), New York: Academic Press.

Ducanis, A. & Golin, A. (1979). *The interdisciplinary health care team: A handbook*. Germantown, MD: Aspen Systems Corporation.

Ephross, P. & Vassil, T. (1987). Towards a model of working groups. *Social Work with Groups, 10*(2), 11-23.

Fessler, S. & Adams, C. (1985). Nurse/social worker role conflict in home health care. *Journal of Gerontological Social Work, 9*(1), 113-123.

Fisher, R. & Ury, W. (1983). *Getting to yes: Negotiating agreement without giving in*. New York: Penguin.

Freidson, E. (1970). *Professional dominance: The structure of medical care*. New York: Aldine-Atherton Press.

Gartner, A. (1975). Four professions: How different, how alike. *Social Work, 20*(5), 353-358.

Gouran, D. (1982). *Making decisions in groups: Choices and consequences*. Glenview, IL: Scott, Foresman & Co.

Halstead, L. (1976). Team care in chronic illness—A critical review of the literature. *Archives of Physical Medicine and Rehabilitation, 57*, 507-511.

Hooyman, E. (1984). Team building in the human services. In B. Compton & B. Galaway (Eds.), *Social work processes* (3rd ed.) (pp. 521-541). Homewood, IL: The Dorsey Press.

Hulme, J., Bach, B. & Lewis, J. (1988). Communication between physicians and physical therapists. *Physician Therapy, 68*(1), 26-31.

Huntington, J. (1981). *Social work and general medical practice: Collaboration or conflict*. London: George Allen Unwin.

Joffe, C. (1979). Abortion work: Strains, coping, strategies, policy implications. *Social Work, 24*, 485-490.

Kadushin, A. (1977). *Consultation in social work*. New York: Columbia University Press.

Kahn, A. (1974). Institutional constraints to interprofessional practice. In H. Rehr (Ed.), *Medicine and social work: An exploration in interprofessionalism* (pp. 14-25). New York: Prodist.

Kane, R. (1975). *Interprofessional teamwork*. Syracuse, NY: Syracuse University School of Social Work.

Kane, R. (1980). Multi-disciplinary teamwork in the U.S.: Trends, issues and implications for the social worker. In S. Lonsdale, A. Webb & T. Briggs (Eds.), *Teamwork in the personal social services and health care* (pp. 138-151). London: Croom Helm.

Kerson, T. (1980). *Medical social work: The pre-professional paradox*. New York: Irvington.

Kulys, R. & Davis, M.A. (1987). Nurses and social workers: Rivals in the provision of social services? *Health and Social Work*, *12*(2), 101-112.

Lonergan, E. (1985). *Group intervention: How to begin and maintain groups in medical and psychiatric settings*. New York: Jason Aronson.

Lowe, J. & Herranen, M. (1978). Conflict in teamwork: Understanding roles and relationships. *Social Work in Health Care*, *3*(3), 323-330.

Lowe, J. & Herranen, M. (1981). Understanding teamwork: Another look at the concepts. *Social Work in Health Care*, *7*(2), 1-11.

Mailick, M. & Ashley, A. (1981). Politics of interprofessional collaboration: Challenge to advocacy. *Social Casework*, *62*(3), 131-137.

Maslach, C. (1978). The client role in staff burnout. *Journal of Social Issues*, *34*(4), 111-124.

Mikula, G. & Schwinger, T. (1978). Intermember relations and reward allocation: Theoretical considerations of affects. In H. Brandslatter, J. Davis & H. Schuler (Eds.), *Dynamics of group decisions* (pp. 229-250). Beverly Hills: Sage Publications.

Mizrahi, T. (1986). *Getting rid of patients: Contradictions in the socialization of physicians*. New Brunswick: Rutgers University Press.

Mizrahi, T. & Abramson, J. (1985). Sources of strain between physicians and social workers: Implications for social workers in health care settings. *Social Work in Health Care*, *10*(3), 33-51.

Nagi, S. (1975). Teamwork in health care in the U.S. *Milbank Memorial Quarterly*, *53*(1), 75-91.

Napier, R. & Gershenfeld, M. (1981). *Groups: Theory and experience* (2nd ed.). Boston: Houghton Mifflin.

Nason, F. (1983). Diagnosing the hospital team. *Social Work in Health Care*, *9*(2), 25-45.

New, P.K.M. (1968). An analysis of the concept of team work. *Community Mental Health Journal*, *4*(4), 326-333.

Northen, H. (1988). *Social work with groups* (2nd ed.). New York: Columbia University Press.

Rapoport, L. (1963). Consultation: An overview. In L. Rapoport (Ed.), *Consultation in social work practice* (pp. 7-20). New York: NASW.

Rosenberg, E. & Nitzberg, H. (1980). The clinical social worker becomes a consultant. *Social Work in Health Care*, *5*(3), 305-312.

Scheidel, T. & Crowell, L. (1979). *Discussing and deciding: A desk book for group leaders and members*. New York: Macmillan.

Shulman, L. (1982). *Skills of supervision and staff management*. Itasca, IL: Peacock.

Shulman, L. (1984). *The skills of helping individuals and groups* (2nd ed.). Itasca, IL: Peacock.

Shulman, L. (1987). Consultation. *Encyclopedia of social work*. Silver Springs, MD: NASW.

Siporin, M. (1956). Dual supervision of psychiatric social workers. *Social Work*, *1*, 32-42.

Spencer, E. & Croley, H. (1963). Administrative consultation. In L. Rapoport (Ed.), *Consultation in social work practice* (pp. 51-68). New York: NASW.

Toseland, R., Palmer-Ganeles, J. & Chapman, D. (1986). Teamwork in psychiatric settings. *Social Work, 31*(1), 46-52.

Toseland, R. & Rivas, R. (1984). *An introduction to group work practice.* New York: Macmillan.

Watkins, E., Holland, T. & Ritvo, R. (1976). Improving the effectiveness of program consultation. *Social Work in Health Care, 2*(1), 43-54.

Watt, J. W. (1985). Protective service teams: The social worker as liaison. *Health and Social Work, 10*(3), 191-197.

Weiner, H. (1959). The hospital, the ward, and the patient as clients: Use of the group method. *Social Work, 4*(4), 57-65.

Weissman, H., Epstein, I. & Savage, A. (1983). *Agency based social work: Neglected aspects of clinical practice.* Philadelphia: Temple University Press.

Whittaker, D. (1975). Some conditions for effective work with groups. *British Journal of Social Work, 5*, 423-439.

Zastrow, C. (1989). *Social work with groups* (2nd ed.). Chicago: Nelson/Hall.

Group Work with Inner City Persons with AIDS

Rachel Child

George S. Getzel

SUMMARY. A model for serving inner city poor persons with AIDS through a medical facility is described. The mixed factors of ethnicity, gender, sexual orientation, race and modes of transmission are examined as influences on the group process. Objectives, pre-group planning, formation guidelines, and presenting problems of members are identified. Through case illustrations group issues are used to point out interventive strategies. Because of the shifting demographics of people with AIDS and their families, the group modality provides a vital educative and supportive vehicle to highly disadvantaged persons affected by the disease.

Serving the inner city poor with AIDS represents a major challenge to human service and health providers. Growing numbers of men, women and children are becoming ill from diseases associated with the high prevalences of the Human Immunodeficiency Virus (HIV) in New York City, Newark, Miami, Los Angeles and elsewhere throughout the United States. Poverty, racism and the inadequacy of the present social bureaucracy provision exacerbate the life chances and the absolute well-being of whole families — parents and children who become HIV infected directly and those who must cope with the illnesses and deaths of loved ones.

The Presidential Commission on the HIV Epidemic (1988, p. 11) acknowledged the importance of addressing the psychosocial needs of AIDS patients who are poor and disadvantaged.

Rachel Child, MA, is a social work student and George S. Getzel, DSW, is Professor at School of Social Work, Hunter College, 129 E. 79th Street, New York, NY 10021.

Certain groups of HIV infected patients may have specific
needs which differ from those of other population groups. For
example, an HIV infected woman of childbearing age has special needs for counseling about the morbidity and mortality
risk to herself and a child she may conceive, . . . children with
HIV infection may have absent or ill parents creating unique
needs for social and supportive services; homeless people with
HIV infection need active assistance in finding a home in order
to contend with this difficult illness. . . . All people with HIV
infection have specific cultural and individual needs which
must be respected . . . In addition, health care services, especially education, counseling and support, and respite care
should be available to the families and loved ones of HIV-
infected persons.

We believe the use of AIDS support groups is one of the most
effective means to address the needs of a range of persons with HIV
infection. Support groups can provide emotional support as well as
assist with the provision of practical and material resources. Thus,
such groups help poor and disadvantaged persons with AIDS
(PWAs) to live a more complete and decent life during the course of
their disease. While AIDS support groups originated largely in
community-based agencies serving gay men, a group work model
of service is viable for a broader spectrum of men and women with
AIDS, including persons with histories of intravenous drug use and
their infected kin. Consequently, we will describe the characteristics of the inner city poor population with AIDS; identify a model of
group work service; and, examine specific issues and interventive
approaches of a group work model for inner city PWAs linked to a
health care setting.

INNER CITY PWAs

Inner city persons with AIDS reflect a variety of complicated
demographic variables which are important to understand in approaching their service needs. According to the Centers for Disease
Control (1988), of the 72,766 cumulative diagnosed cases of AIDS
as of September 12, 1988, 63% were gay or bisexual men; 19%

intravenous drug users; 7% were gay men with a history of intravenous drug use; 3% were persons judged to be infected through heterosexual contact; and, the remaining 9% were persons judged to be infected by blood transfusions, blood products or from unknown origins.

The inner city population with AIDS is reflected in national statistics. Black and Hispanic PWAs were 26% and 15%, respectively, of all cumulative cases, and white non-Hispanic and Asian/Pacific Islanders, 59% and 1% respectively. Among male intravenous drug users without a history of homosexuality, 38% were Black and 44% were Hispanic. Twenty-two percent of all intravenous drug users with AIDS were women; or 53% of all women with AIDS, a large proportion of whom were inner city Black and Hispanic women. Twenty-seven percent of all women with AIDS were infected by males with a history of intravenous drug use or homosexual behaviors; 65% of these women were Black and 11% Hispanic. Of children with AIDS infected before or at birth by their mothers, approximately 61% were Black and 24% Hispanic.

For example, New York City is overwhelmed with the impact of AIDS on entire families. As of April 1988, New York City had 293 (31%) of the nation's pediatric AIDS cases (children under the age 13); of these, 72% were associated with intravenous drug use in one or both parents. Thus, the proportion of intravenous drug AIDS cases in New York City continues to grow, with its disproportionate effects on the poor and on minorities (New York City, 1988).

Honey (1988, p. 365) notes the important role of the hospital providing care for the inner city family affected by AIDS because ". . . ethnic minority populations . . . frequently support families on incomes barely above the poverty levels. Many must survive on public assistance." The hospital staff and social work staff of hospitals coordinate medical and social welfare services in a form unavailable outside that one institution. The social workers in hospitals are also expert in obtaining funds for service payment.

For inner city persons with HIV infections and AIDS, the stresses on their extant material and emotional supports are enormous. In order to alleviate these stresses a major effort at outreach and education about the available resources of formal providers like hospitals and public assistance agencies is required. Case management and advocacy by social workers become crucial functions in developing necessary services, including the provision of group work services (Napoleone, 1988; Sonsel, Paradise, & Stroup, 1988; and Lewart, 1988).

TOWARD A GROUP WORK MODEL

According to Gambe and Getzel (in press) an AIDS support group represents an optimizing service strategy when it cogwheels with requisite individual crisis services, entitlement advocacy and informational and referral services. A group work service also must be able to help group members with issues of support from kin and friends as well as assistance from health care, income maintenance, and social service organizations.

A group work model appropriate for work with inner city PWAs must give primacy to empowerment of the clients (Haney, 1988). Workers must constantly acknowledge the changing needs and wants of the membership who frequently feel powerless and out of control because of their illnesses and the vicissitudes of their changing environments. A group work approach to PWAs should simultaneously focus on those biopsychosocial crises that are time limited as well as engage the membership, for however long they are in the group, in problem-solving. This mutual aid process helps group members to deal with the common and shared aspects of the experience of living with AIDS and its social and existential isolation. Strong group cohesion and the expression of powerful emotions follow in rapid succession as individuals and the group together face new symptoms, medical procedures, and loss as well as periods of hope and the expression of love and caring in and outside the group. Historic issues of family conflict, loss, and guilt over past wrongs may also become subjects of group discussion.

The efforts of group workers with PWAs focus on the following objectives (Gambe and Getzel, in press):

1. Identifying ways to reach out to families, friends and others for practical and emotional support during periods of illness and hospitalization;
2. Expressing otherwise unacceptable feelings of rage, sadness,

jealousy, shame, and guilt occasioned by biopsychosocial crises;

3. Identifying ways to counter bouts of acute death anxiety occasioned by the recognition of personal mortality;

4. Exploring quality of life options (how people want to live and
die) as they grow more dependent on health and social service
providers for their care;

5. Finding practical ways to live hopefully and affirmatively day
by day;

6. Finding ways to demonstrate concern for peers, family and
friends who themselves may be overwhelmed by illness;

7. Examining methods to leave a legacy that connotes the mean-
ings of their lives after death;

8. Constructing a personal belief system and group ideology that
reinforce members' positive self-worth despite rebukes and
hurt to be found all about them.

GROUP PLANNING AND FORMATION

In planning a PWA support group linked to a health care organization, or one that has hospital support, the workers must, of necessity, be flexible. Through experience with groups in an inner city
hospital, the authors have determined that group membership is
much less homogenized than a traditional group therapy model due
to the nature of the referral process from doctors and other health
care professionals. Because the group is for support, all persons
newly diagnosed with AIDS should be allowed to attend. The initial
shock, dismay and sense of stigmatization of the newly diagnosed
AIDS patient are often lessened if he or she realizes that the group is
for all PWAs, no matter what their background or current state of
health.

The intake interview of new members, therefore, is largely to
determine a person's mental state rather than an attempt to weed out
those of dissimilar background. Some prospective members may be
affected by AIDS dementia, drug use, or current drug withdrawal
and would therefore be unsuitable for a support group, unless they
are also undergoing therapy for those conditions. The intake inter-

view should also determine if the person has a sufficient ability to speak English, or the common group language, to understand the other group members. Finally, the intake interview serves to explain to prospective members the nature of a support group, and to determine if the individual is willing to join in the group process. The fact that the group will always be there to support the member, no matter what the state of his or her health and no matter what his or her social background is, cannot be stressed enough.

As stated by Gambe and Getzel (in press), it is essential that there be co-leadership of the group. This provides greater assurance that the group will meet each week at a regular time, offering the membership a sense of stability and continued support. Co-leadership also enables the group leaders to give each other additional emotional support, badly needed when working with terminally ill patients. This is particularly true when working with AIDS patients as the course of the illness is not predictable, and as many of the opportunistic infections are physically disfiguring in the extreme. Workers must develop a tolerance for accepting the ravages of the illness. Co-workers also need to gain support from each other because of the strain produced by working with a group with members who come from different ethnic, racial and social class backgrounds.

If possible, the support group should meet in a hospital location accessible to those in wheelchairs and to those undergoing (portable) infusion therapy. It should also be easily accessible to outpatients who return to the hospital for group sessions. The meeting place should not be labelled as a part of an AIDS unit, so that outpatients are not further stigmatized. The room should be warm as AIDS patients are often exceptionally thin and suffer from temperature change. Smoking should not be allowed and the ventilation should be good so that those recovering from pneumonia or using supplementary oxygen have the cleanest possible air.

Once the group has started, a decision should be taken by its members as to general rules. These would cover such subjects as the number of new members to be admitted at one meeting time, what to do about lateness, a determination if there should be disclosure of telephone numbers and addresses and the necessity for confidentiality. The initial membership should be involved in as much of this contracting as possible as the process is empowering and gives a sense of control. Workers should, however, be specific about hospital regulations and should introduce new members, as they join the group, to the group's contracted rules.

The following descriptions of members of an inner city hospital PWA group reflect the characteristic mix of gender, racial, ethnic and social backgrounds:

Z. is a white male, age 50. He has a college education and is currently in graduate school. He is a former IV drug user, was married and has a son who lives abroad. He has an enormous wealth of information about the medical aspects of AIDS and reads voraciously on the subject in scientific journals. Z. has enthusiasm for and knowledge of new drug therapies and is convinced he will live long enough to "lick this thing." When the subjects discussed in the group become emotional, he will usually try and switch them back to the more scientific aspects of the disease or intellectualize his responses. He is stocky and holds his body rigidly, yet gestures wildly with his hands. Z. was diagnosed 15 months ago.

A. is a black male, age 29. He is homosexual and was a male prostitute. A man of outrageous humor and wit, he tends to dominate the meetings with dramatic renditions of his current relationships to the medical establishment, his friends and his family. He invariably talks too long and is too loud, but can also be very kindly and supportive of fellow group members. He is emaciated and weak, but has a very loud voice and uses his large hands in extravagant poses. He was diagnosed nine months ago.

L. is a racial and ethnic mixture of Anglo, Black, and Hispanic. She is 38. She has two children and was married twice. Her first husband was an IV drug user. Her second husband died of AIDS. She is the "mother" of the group and does a great deal of networking between group members outside the hospital setting. Something of an authority on homeopathic remedies, she also has a wealth of information about the hospital's medical staff, procedures for obtaining various experimental drugs, and continually stresses that AIDS patients must take control of their treatment and must be positive. L. is very beautiful and very healthy looking. She radiates compassion and kindness. She has been a member of the group for two years.

M. is an Hispanic female, age 40. She was a narcotics addict from age 14 to age 35. She had one child when she was 20 who was taken from her at age six months by the Bureau of Child Welfare. She has lost contact with that child. Her second child was shot in a drug related gang war when he was 10. It was at this point that M. gave up drugs and joined Narcotics Anonymous. She became a group leader and finally a paid staff member of that organization. She is very short, very stocky, sits up very straight and punches at the air as she talks. M. has been diagnosed for three months.

P. is a 35-year-old Anglo bisexual. He is married, but has no children. His wife does not know of his diagnosis. He comes from a very conservative and large extended family. He has worked in hospitals most of his life and is very knowledgeable about hospital and medical politics. P. is very good looking and flirtatious, very well dressed and is optimistic about his current health. Having been diagnosed four years ago, he says, "I lived the longest in this group and so I got a lot to say about your attitude. It's gotta be good to survive."

After the group is established, membership will often wish to engage in their own selection process, in spite of the "open" nature of the group, in cooperation with the social worker. PWA group members and social workers often are concerned with the behavior of new members who are attending. For example, some new members may be suffering dementia. Others may still be on drugs, and not able to relate to the group. In the most extreme cases, a member with a new diagnosis may be on drugs, slightly demented and too hostile to be able to relate to others. This group concern is sometimes verbalized and sometimes not. Furthermore, there are times when the social worker may decide that a member should not be allowed back in the group because of inappropriate behavior. When concerns about members' behavior arise, both the group members and the social workers need to have cooperative roles in the process of determining who should and who should not be allowed in the group, and, the social worker may need to guide decision making. At other times, very sick members may be difficult for the group to accept for a variety of physical and/or psychological reasons. The following is an illustration of such a group reaction.

A core group member, C., had been deteriorating . . . He was in a wheelchair and continually coughed up sputum that was bloody. He would spit this into a paper cup which sometimes slipped out of his trembling hands. Other group members would look away, or make high signs to each other. He began to show signs of dementia, not making connections at times and rambling on, interrupting. C. was, however, one of the oldest members of the group and would, from time to time, be lucid. The social worker felt C. should be a member of the group if at all possible, because he had contributed so much in the past. The social worker also felt that he was too sick to be there and caused a reactive process that was disruptive of the group. Furthermore the social worker realized that she wished to protect the group and herself from the total deterioration that AIDS can bring. C. had been the poet of the group, and she hated to see that part of him gone.

At the next group meeting, when C. was not present, Z. started off immediately saying that he had something to say, that would probably sound nasty, but that he just had to say it. He said he just couldn't stand having to sit and worry if that "Goddamned cup of C.'s" would slip and spill again. This was the opening wedge and the group reacted by howling with laughter, and admission that it had bothered them all. L., the group mother, said "It's so hard to see him so very sick and he just doesn't make sense any more." A. said, "You know, folks, when I look at him, I see what can happen to me. And, in God's love, if you drop me when I'm like that, I'll kill you all . . . because if I think you're all I got now, you'll REALLY be all that I got then." The group responded with "Amen" and sudden laughter, in relief that an unspoken vote had been taken. (C. came to only one more group where he was cared for tenderly by the membership. He died a week later.)

GROUP COMMONALITIES AND DIFFERENCES

In this type of group for PWAs the most obvious commonality is that all its members have AIDS. They all have a sword of Damocles hanging over their heads. It is a double edged sword in that they wait for the next opportunistic infection, as well as for eventual death. Group members function individually in one or another stage of denial, anger, bargaining, depression or acceptance (Kubler-Ross, 1969) of their mortality. These stages come and go, not necessarily in order, depending on the state of physical and psychological health of the individual member and on his or her social support base. The emotional instability that PWA group members experience can be illustrated by the following:

O. walked into the group and said that he couldn't see too well and that he was angry with the doctors because they weren't helping him. This inspired B. who spoke of his anger that the drug DHPG (used to treat an opportunistic infection) hadn't helped him and in a rage described being injected in the eyeballs with that drug. Then S. jumped in and said that when he was admitted to a hospital in Westchester, he spent 56 hours in an emergency room and then nobody would touch him. As he said this he punched his hand into his fist and banged on an adjacent chair. Z. said that he felt that really only a small minority of doctors were useless. S. interrupted him and said "Fuck this shit. I wanted and needed someone to help me!" The social worker then asked the group what they did generally with this kind of rage. S. again spoke and said, "I feel like, today, I'm on a roller coaster of emotion. I can't control it; I'm out of control." T. said that he was, too, at times and spoke of his blinding rage at a friend who was still having unsafe sex, and of how he tried to beat him up. B. said that he gets angry at those closest to him, but never cries. "I'm just bitchy and horrible." L. said it *was* like a roller coaster and, turning to S., said, "Accept those ups and downs. That's you

now. You are going up and down. Your body's doing it as
well as your head.''

In our experience, the membership usually has a common referral
base in that they are using the same hospital, medical team and
community resources. Most inner city PWA group members using
the same hospital come from the same community and are aware of
what community reaction to their diagnosis would be. Most members of inner city groups are poor. A number of them have children.
A majority of those parents are single parents. PWA mothers and
fathers are concerned that their children's futures be secure. Therefore, most do not tell their children that they have AIDS.

> If I tell my kid or anybody that I got AIDS, it'll get out. And
> you know what'll happen in that school. They'll beat up on
> him. No sir, NOBODY at that school's going to know. And
> my kid ain't going to know. I'll not lay that one on him. Hav-
> ing your father die is bad enough.

In families where one of several children may also have AIDS or
be HIV infected, the PWA parent faces an additional stressor.

> Who's going to take my children when I go? He (the child's
> father) wants to take the one who's OK. I don't want my kids
> split up! They're a family. They need each other. It's not right
> to split up a family.

Brought up in the inner city with restricted opportunities, many
members may have had little experience with significant task completion. Because many of the IV drug users escape into the drug
culture in early adolescence, their identities may be shaky. If they
have had limited success in mastering developmental transitions,
they may not be prepared to cope with such a change in life circum-
stance (Erikson, 1975).

> R. said she was so tired. She'd been discharged from the
> hospital the week before and celebrated by going out dancing.
> A. said, ''. . . and I'll bet you took something that helped you
> get yourself that energy too.'' R. petulantly said that she didn't
> see why she couldn't have a bit of fun once in a while, that

she was tired to death of being a "Fuckin' good girl." L. responded by saying that if she kept up abusing her body, she was going to be a "Fucking dead girl sooner than you should." R. said, "But that's how I always have fun."

Hispanic and West Indian PWAs may become frustrated in their attempts to be responsive to two, sometimes conflicting cultures (Sewell-Coker, Hamilton-Collins, & Fein, 1985).

N. speaks of his confusion. His large and extended family has bonded together to protect him. "My God, they don't want me to do anything without them. They don't even want me to go to the doctor or to see my friends. It's like I was back in the village in P.R. again. I feel like I'm suffocating with all this goddamned love. It's like I can do nothin' on my own no more. It's like they're taking away what's left of me."

After an AIDS diagnosis, members initially come to a group in a state of enormous bewilderment and emotional upheaval. When their development has been complicated by dual cultural expectations, as mentioned above, this sense of displacement and emotional turmoil is magnified. Although the worker needs to be aware of how cultural factors may influence members' response to AIDS, usually cultural differences are overcome by the commonality of the disease experience. All PWA group members will feel stigmatized by the disease. They are isolated by their society and, in some instances, by their families. The isolation is particularly felt by those who have minimal education, who know little of the disease, and whose neighbors, friends and families are terrified of contagion.

B. walked into the group. He was pouting. He said "I can't go home to my island. I will be shunned there. They are terrified of AIDS. And I just came from my doctor and he uses rubber gloves when he touches me. I feel so alone. I want hugs. I just want someone to touch me."

Since inner city groups for PWAs are typically composed of a mix of Black, Hispanic, and Anglo members, the social worker should be sensitive to behavior in the group that may stem from

ethnic identification. Certainly, cultural or ethnic "styles" can affect how members behave. Social workers should accept these behavioral variations but be wary of making generalizations.

GROUP ISSUES

It is interesting to observe that, no matter what the patient composition of any group, the dynamic of each group meeting is approximately the same. There is a distinctive developmental cycle: a
self-initiated cohesive phase, a triggered emotional outburst or tran-
sition phase, and then a stronger re-bonding or grouping at the end
after the emotional response has been accepted and worked through
by the group. Each meeting encompasses some of the group development steps described by Garland (Garland, Jones, & Kolodny,
1973).

Once the meeting has started, and business is discussed, there is
usually a silence which is immediately broken by one of the more
educated and articulate members. He or she will bring up a safe
subject, one that can elicit a general group response of agreement.
This will most often be a reaction to a television program or news-
paper article in which AIDS is discussed, and which offended the
member initiating the discussion. Usually a certain amount of group
rage is articulated as in the following example.

> "I saw the Oprah show and, man, I was disgusted. Terrible!
> Did you hear that? (General nodding and lots of "yeahs.")
> And did you see that audience and they don't know *nothing*
> about what it's about. They were bigots!" (There was general
> agreement in response to the statement. Then, other TV shows
> were mentioned that had offended, and a certain amount of
> generalized rage was let go.)

The group thereby re-bonds by challenging the stigma and social
isolation caused by their common diagnosis. Once they feel comfortable in their commonality, the members can start to work. Common subjects discussed in the work phase of each meeting are:

1. Stigmatization and reactions from neighbors, family, friends, doctors and dentists. The isolation that results from that stigmatization. The need to be silent.
2. The need for education about transmission. How to convince others that it is difficult to get AIDS. Others' fear of touching a patient, of sharing food or dishes with them, and the resultant anger this produces in group members.
3. Sexuality and "safer sex." The loss of libido. How to tell, and *if* you tell, sex partners of your diagnosis.
4. Taking charge of your own medication. Learning to observe and trust your own bodily response to medication. Being positive and forceful and, in some instances, oppositional to doctors and to hospital staff.
5. Projection of anger and acceptance of that anger by the group.
6. Giving each other support in and out of the hospital. Caring for each other.

During this work phase, there is rarely disagreement and support is given quite openly. The work is, by and large, that of an individual's expressing his or her own concerns and feelings about one of the above topics. The group members' response is two-fold: they accept the member's concern and feeling, and if possible, try to support the feeling and to resolve the concern. The basic contract of the group is, therefore, one of giving support and help.

In spite of variations in style of emotional response, group members avoid personal conflict. As former IV drug users, possibly from poor, Black, white or Hispanic communities, or of a homosexual sexual persuasion, they have often been labeled as outsiders prior to their diagnosis. This fragile identity is usually further fragmented by an AIDS diagnosis. One can appreciate the group's need to stay at a support level (Lonergan, 1980) and attempts to try to solidify intra-group connectedness.

> When asked by a social worker how he managed to get along with such a mixed group of people, of people who were not as educated as he, W. responded, "Sister, you just don't get it. It's like we're all in this foxhole together. We've *got* to stay together. Because, at the moment, that's all we've got. Each other."

At the end of each group there are usually tension relieving moments of humor, an exchange of medical information and another re-bonding by a generalized complaint against "the system," similar to the initial group bonding, and possibly by a closing ritual initiated when the group was formed. For example, members kiss and embrace one another.

ROLE OF WORKERS

The social workers serve four functions within an AIDS support group: (1) They help to lead the group, encouraging acceptance of individual members' often highly varied emotional processes by the rest of the group, enabling the group to deal with common issues and problem solve; (2) They help patients resolve specific concrete extra-hospital needs; (3) They encourage the group members to act as their own social workers, to solve their own problems, and to regain a sense of control over their own lives; and (4) They are members of the group, expressing their own emotional response and becoming involved in the supporting process, thereby lessening the patients' fear of the medical or social work institution and lessening the patients' sense of stigmatization.

There is an acceptance of the fragility of the individual, and an almost stated need not to rock the boat that is the group. The group gives its individual members support and an acceptable identity which they badly need. AIDS patients suffer both ego and bodily damage (Gambe & Getzel, in press). They are constantly concerned about their immediate and future survival needs. Added to this must be the differences among individuals, in social and ethnic background, which make it difficult to communicate at some levels. For these reasons, certain potentially conflictual subjects related to individual differences are rarely mentioned in the group; the tendency for a rivalry between gay members and the IV drug users, between Black and Hispanic, and between men and women are usually not discussed. Further, older group members tend to feel that the newer members do not understand yet what it is like to live with AIDS. Although death is rarely mentioned, it remains a shadow on all group members. Members embrace one another as if to ward off the eventuality of death and more separation.

Inner city patients are similar to other AIDS patients. They are concerned with living with AIDS. They wish to live as best they can. In order to do this, however, they must have additional support and care because of the complexity of their environmental situation, individual differences related to their cultural and ethnic background and societal stigmatization. A hospital or social service institution support group of this type can help, by its very nature, to rebuild shattered identities, and thereby provide that support and care.

REFERENCES

Centers for Disease Control. (September 1988). *AIDS weekly surveillance report.* Atlanta, Georgia: Centers for Disease Control.

Gambe, R. & Getzel, G. (in press). Group Work with gay persons with AIDS. *Social Casework.*

Garland, J.A., Jones, H.E. & Kolodny, R.L., (1973). A model for stages of development in social work groups. In S. Bernstein (Ed). *Explorations in group work* (pp. 17-71). Boston: Milford House.

Haney, P. (1988). Providing empowerment to the person with AIDS. *Social Work, 33* (pp. 251-253).

Honey, E. (1988). AIDS in the inner city. *Social Casework, 69* (pp. 365-370).

Howard, A. & Scott, R.A. (1981). The study of minority groups in complex societies. In R. Munroe and Associates (Eds.), *Handbook of cross-cultural human development* (pp. 113-149). New York: Garland STPM Press.

Kubler-Ross, E. (1969). *On death and dying.* New York: Macmillan.

Lewart, G. (1988). Children and AIDS. *Social Casework, 69* (pp. 349-354).

Lonergan, E.C. (1988). Humanizing the hospital experience: Report of a group for medical patients. *Health and Social Work, 6* (pp. 533-63).

New York Intra-agency Task Force on AIDS (May 1988). *New York City Strategic Plan for AIDS.* New York: City of New York.

Presidential Commission on the Human Immunodeficiency Virus. (June 1988). The report of the President's Commission. Washington, DC: U.S. Government Printing Office.

Sewell-Coker, B., Hamilton-Collins, J. & Fein, E. (1985). Social work practice with West Indian immigrants. *Social Casework, 66* (pp. 563-568).

Sonsel, G.E., Paradise, F. & Stroup, S. (1988). Case management practice in an AIDS service organization. *Social Casework, 69* (pp. 388-392).

Wilson, G. (1976). From practice to theory: a personalized history. In Roberts, R.W. and Northern, H. (Eds.), *Theories of social work with groups* (pp. 1-44). New York: Columbia University Press.

Self-Help Groups:
An Empowerment Vehicle
for Sickle Cell Disease Patients
and Their Families

Kermit B. Nash

SUMMARY. The results of a national survey on self-help groups for individuals and families where sickle cell anemia exist will be described. Data were gathered on the type of self-help groups, goals, membership, frequency of meetings, relationships with professionals and services rendered. Study results suggest that these self-help groups play a major role in empowerment for individuals and their families where this disease exists.

Patients who have sickle cell disease, like all patients who have a chronic illness or disability, are disempowered because of features associated with the disease state. Sickle Cell Disease, a group of inherited disorders of the red blood cells characterized by chronic anemia, results from a defect in the metabolism of hemoglobin. The disease primarily, but not exclusively, affects Blacks. Individuals with Sickle Cell Disease are reported to have a high incidence of poor personal and social adjustment and display significant stressful impacts on family functioning (Nishiura, Whitten & Jenkins, 1980; Vavasseur, 1977). These problems are intensified by the lack of adequate information and counseling, by the varying quality of medical facilities and by the increased financial and emotional demands made on the families, all of which frequently foster an attitude of helplessness. Other features that have been identified as

Kermit B. Nash, PhD, is affiliated with the School of Social Work, University of North Carolina at Chapel Hill, Chapel Hill, NC 27599-3550.

81

disempowering for individuals with a chronic disease or disability like sickle cell disease include: limitations in physical functioning and restraints on roles and abilities; inappropriate reaction and actions of others; passivity demanded by the patient role; and, inequitable actions of community institutions (Antonovsky, 1980; Chesler & Barbarin, 1986; Chesler & Chesney, 1988; Featherstone, 1980; Taylor, 1979).

Self-help groups can serve as a mechanism for reversing the process of disempowerment. The support, education, counseling and advocacy available in self-help groups offer the individual and family the means to achieve empowerment and "to take charge of their lives." Self-help groups for sickle cell disease patients can empower their members by allowing individuals to contribute to the welfare of others with a similar condition and by encouraging them to mobilize themselves and others for action and change (Chesler & Chesney, 1988). Unfortunately, there is virtually no research and little descriptive information available on self-help groups for sickle cell patients and their families.

The purpose of this paper is to consider the potential of self-help groups for empowering sickle cell patients and their families; and, to report the findings of a national survey of self-help groups for individuals with Sickle Cell Disease. This represents a pilot effort to explore systematically how self-help groups are being used by this population. Data will be presented on types of self-help groups identified, group membership, frequency of meetings, group relations with professionals, services rendered and goals of these groups.

EMPOWERMENT

Empowerment is a key social and psychological construct that is directly linked to a person's ability to function effectively within the immediate family system and the larger society. For individuals with chronic and disabling conditions, such as Sickle Cell Disease, and their families, empowerment has special meaning. For the patient, it means having the capacity for self-care, knowing when and at what point medical care should be sought, and establishing a positive self-concept and identity. For families, it means greater clarity about family roles, the capacity to provide effective care for ill family members, and the ability to treat episodes of crisis without specific interventions by medical professionals. Further, for both patients and families, empowerment represents the capacity to be proactive on behalf of self and the community (Chesler & Chesney, 1988). Such a proactive stance includes the dissemination of appropriate knowledge about Sickle Cell Disease to promote understanding of the range of functioning of people with the disease and their service needs. Increasingly, members of self-help groups are participating in the education of professionals in hospital grand rounds and educational activities for school personnel.

Solomon (1976) conceptualizes empowerment as a helping approach focused on the relationship between those who have power and those who are powerless. Powerlessness manifests itself at both the individual and societal level. On the individual level those who have Sickle Cell Disease may incorporate into their developmental experience a negative valuation of themselves. This population is stigmatized both by their minority status and by the chronic disease which can affect their ability to function effectively. Further, Sickle Cell Disease may result in limited interpersonal and educational development which reinforces the individual's (and family's) inability to handle problems which arise and to effectively navigate institutions offering services. Society, through misinformation and discrimination, frequently reinforces inadequacy by the denial of employment or the limited funding of programs to serve this population.

Toseland and Hacker (1982) report that professionals perform important functions in supporting the growth and continued existence of self-help groups. Professionals support, initiate and develop self-help groups in a variety of settings and coordinate their activities with self-help groups. Helping professionals also serve as advocates, negotiators, facilitators and advisors in formal and informal systems. Their focus is on creating a climate that promotes the development of members' personal resources such as positive self-concept, cognitive skills, knowledge, health and physical competence. These personal resources lead to the development of interpersonal, technical, and organizational skills that will enhance the social functioning and problem solving skills of their members (Paz, 1986).

Self-help groups can be considered empowering because they

promote processes and practices that encourage personal disclosure and networking. They create opportunities for sharing emotional experiences and allow individuals to gain access to information, new coping skills and practical resources. The exchange of information and concerns can be beneficial to both members and guests. This is frequently true of meetings with physicians. Visits by physicians give members an opportunity to have an exchange with medical professionals outside of clinical settings. The atmosphere tends to be more relaxed than in the hospital or clinic, a factor which tends to decrease the anxiety level of the members. It is not uncommon for the identification and resolution of problems in the health care delivery system to emerge from the self-help group process. For example, one Sickle Cell self-help group organized, networked and protested emergency room care offered to family members. Representatives of the group approached hospital administrators with their concerns. As a result, the group was invited to participate in the development of protocol for the handling of Sickle Cell Disease patients seen in the emergency room.

SICKLE CELL DISEASE

Sickle Cell Anemia is an hereditary, hematologic disorder for which there is no known cure. Treatment is symptomatic and palliative in nature. There can be both medical and non-medical complications. While the disease primarily affects people of African descent, the gene for Sickle hemoglobin is found among populations adjacent to the Mediterranean Sea and Indian Ocean. These groups include Italians, Greeks, Yugoslavians, Western Asians, Turks, Southern Iranians, Indo-Chinese, and American Indians. Due to the lack of effective screening programs, no accurate statistics are available as to its frequency among the total susceptible population. Data has become available for the frequency of Sickle Cell Anemia, the most common form of Sickle Cell Disease among Black populations in the United States, with the advent of federally funded community screening programs. Its prevalence among Blacks varies widely, according to the literature. The best estimate of Sickle Cell Anemia occurrences for Blacks is 1 in 625 (0.17%) (Motulsky, 1973).

The signs and symptoms of Sickle Cell Disease are myriad, as would be suspected from a disease that produces its symptoms on the basis of an obstructed blood flow. The disorder begins at birth and lasts throughout the life span of the individual which now, not infrequently, extends into the fourth or fifth decades, and in some instances even longer. Virtually any tissue or organ may be affected (Smith, 1983). Some of the major problems include: infection in the young, strokes, sickle cell retinopathy in adolescents, and aseptic necrosis of bones in adults. There is a significant increase in morbidity and mortality for pregnant women, priaprism in men, use of transfusion therapy and painful crises (Smith, 1983). The frequency and the severity of the crises are unpredictable but they can be painful and of long duration.

PSYCHOSOCIAL IMPLICATIONS

The psychosocial effects of sickle cell disease are similar to those for any other chronic disease. Like other hereditary diseases, Sickle Cell Disease has its primary impact on the individual whose physical abilities are impaired, who is in pain, and whose life expectancy may be shortened. Further, the fact that the disease primarily affects Blacks has exacerbated problems associated with this chronic condition. The fear and suspicion, raised in the Black community by perceived and real discrimination in employment and insurance coverage, add to the physical pain associated with the disease. Since the mid-seventies this so-called "killer disease" has been making sensational copy for newspapers and television shows. Some Blacks have apparently regarded this publicity about the disease with shame and suspicion and claimed that it provided racists with new ammunition to degrade members of the Black race further (Scott, 1983).

Psychosocial factors associated with Sickle Cell Disease have an influence on individual aspirations and family dynamics. These include social, psychological, economic, legal and interpersonal factors. Problems are intensified by the lack of adequate information and counseling, by the varying quality of medical facilities and the fragmentation of services (Alleyne & Sergeant, 1976; Battle, 1984;

Evans, Burlew & Oler, 1988; Whitten & Fischoff, 1974; Williams, Earles & Pack, 1983).

The specific psychosocial implications concern the physical limitations, the reaction of others, and the internal reactions that cause stress. The impact of unpredictable and painful episodes may manifest in impaired self-esteem, helplessness, fear and poor self-concept (Conyard, Krishnamurthy & Dosile, 1980). Growth retardation, delayed onset of puberty, the fact that there is no cure, frequent hospitalizations, and teasing by others can exacerbate the psychosocial damage. Due to their physical limitations, older patients may have been shattered in their youth. Thus, they may not only lack the prerequisite skills to achieve successful employment, but also may have little or no knowledge about the world (Johnson, 1981). It is not uncommon to meet young adults who have dropped out of school and are unprepared for adult life because they have been told they would not live to be an adult.

Adults are concerned about decreased life expectancy, marriage, pregnancy, and lessened vitality. Patients may have valid worries about such basic economic needs as continuation of disability payments, transportation, and housing. These anxieties influence decisions about medical care and involvement with a comprehensive rehabilitation program. Further, all of these concerns continue to be compounded by the adverse effects of legislation in the early seventies (Scott, 1983). In that era, misguided but well intentioned individuals began mass screening programs; legislators rushed to push for legislation, mandatory testing; fraudulent benefit promoters and bogus organizations emerged; and, some leaders advised Blacks to refuse screening that might lead to loss of jobs and insurance coverage (Scott, 1983). Because of individual and familial concerns that are reinforced by negative community and societal reactions, the patient and family may view themselves negatively, experiencing disempowerment and considerable stress.

Stress indicators in families with Sickle Cell Disease have been identified. These include the severe pain of some crises, the unpredictability of onset, the threat of imminent death, the fear of some siblings that it can "happen to them," the chronicity and the limited medical management techniques available at present. Most of the resources are focused on patient treatment and there has been little attention to providing family support. Education about the disease tends to be inadequate and service delivery is fragmented (Chamberlain, Nash & Woodward, 1974; Nash, 1986; Williams, 1983).

The reactions of others in the community may increase the disempowerment of patients and their families. Parents are often overprotective as they try to prevent recurrences of painful episodes in children and adolescents. These attempts are further compounded by the guilt that surrounds the hereditary nature of the illness. Affected children are often given an inaccurate prognosis of a shortened life span, which may decrease their motivation to achieve and encourages family members to foster dependency. The educational deficits and poor school performance which may result from excessive absenteeism can add to disempowerment. Further, in many cases, employers who are reluctant to hire sickle cell patients and who discriminate against them reinforce disempowerment. Incidents of discrimination range from high school graduates who were given high grades, but can't read, to airlines denying employment (which was later challenged successfully in court).

The internalized reactions to the stresses associated with Sickle Cell Disease can cause anger, resentment, hostility, depression, hopelessness, helplessness, weak ego, guilt, anxiety, frustration, self-pity, denial, and over-compensation. Self-help groups can serve as a vehicle to offset reactions to stress and facilitate the empowerment process. Although professional counseling and family support services may be helpful, self-help groups for sickle cell patients and their families provide both tangible and intangible support in a way that empowers members. They offer information, opportunity for skill development and advocacy as well as the reassurance of shared experiences. Self-help groups serve as a focal point for community participation, provide an opportunity to develop leadership skills, and offer experiences which raise self-esteem.

SICKLE CELL DISEASE SELF-HELP GROUPS

As noted earlier, self-help groups are viewed by professional health workers as an emerging social resource that provides support for children and families with a variety of health conditions. Among the benefits of this support are education, coping, self-actualization, advocacy and empowerment (Black & Drachman, 1985; Katz, 1980; Lurie & Shulman, 1983). Although no empirical studies dealing with self-help groups and Sickle Cell Anemia have been reported in the literature, self-help groups for genetic diseases and genetic blood disorders have been described since the 1950s. Katz (1984) noted the following advantages of self-help groups for genetic blood disorders:

1. provide social support and decrease feelings of isolation;
2. provide practical information and resources that enable patients, families, and relatives to better understand the problems associated with genetic disorders;
3. allow a greater sense of autonomy and decision making, thereby decreasing dependency;
4. overcome the stigma and discrimination associated with illness, disability, and other physical and mental disorders;
5. enhance communication among members of the self-help groups and helping professionals including physicians, therapists, nurses, social workers, and vocational counselors and people who deal with related problems, such as housing and legal issues; and,
6. advocate the provision and delivery of services as well as necessary research and training programs.

In recent years, several accounts of the use of self-help groups by sickle cell patients, family and significant others to supplement services have appeared in the literature (Corley, 1986; Evans, 1983, 1985). Further, J. Vavasseur, Director of Program Development for the National Association for Sickle Cell Disease, Inc., has reported that information collected by the Association indicates their twenty-seven affiliates have self-help groups (personal communications, July 24, 1985). The purposes of self-help groups for sickle cell patients and their families appear to be somewhat diffuse. Some groups are designed for education, while some are for recreation, others for advocacy and empowerment (Corley, 1986; Evans, 1985).

Early reports of self-help groups for sickle cell patients and their families represent impressions of a particular group or statements from panels at conferences composed of self-help members from different groups in a given geographical area. Informal reports on such groups throughout the country were shared at the First National Conference on Self-Help Groups for Genetic Blood Disorder held in Washington, DC in June 1984. These anecdotal reports highlighted the fact that little is known about self-help groups for patients with Sickle Cell Disease and their families. The individual reports stressed the benefits of self-help groups for individuals affected with the disease and their families and emphasized the need to know more about self-help groups for this population. There was no systematic information on how many such groups existed, how often they met, who were the members, whether professionals were involved or not, what the group goals were and the effectiveness of these groups.

STUDY DESIGN

A survey of activities in sickle cell self-help group settings was conducted to obtain information about how self-help groups were being used for sickle cell patients and their families. In order to reach as many sickle cell groups and organizations as possible a self-administered questionnaire was distributed at the Ninth Annual Comprehensive Sickle Cell Centers meeting held in Los Angeles, California on March 11-12, 1985. This questionnaire was completed by the 36 staff members in attendance at the meeting who were from seven Sickle Cell Clinics, Sickle Cell Centers, and twenty Sickle Cell Associations.

The questionnaire, consisting of 16 closed and open-ended questions, was designed to determine the existence and extent of such groups for sickle cell patients, to describe the services provided to group members, and to elicit answers regarding group goals, structure and processes. These questions were asked to explore anecdotal accounts about how self-help groups served to empower members.

RESULTS

Twenty-nine of the 36 respondents identified at least one sickle cell self-help group. Two of the larger centers reported two groups. While seven respondents indicated that their organization did not have or support a self-help group, five of these seven respondents reported organizational plans to start a self-help group in the near future.

Purpose

Since reports of self-help groups for sickle cell patients and their families note a variety of purposes, the questionnaire requested information about the type, or purpose, of the group. The 29 respondents characterized the purposes of their self-help groups by checking one or more of the following categories: (a) Behavioral control; (b) Common stressful predicament; (c) Survival orientation; (d) Personal growth; and (e) Enhance effectiveness in daily living. Eighteen (62%) reported that their groups were designed to enhance effectiveness in daily living. Thirteen respondents (45%) reported groups were focused on personal growth. Ten respondents (34%) reported that groups provided relief from a common stressful predicament. Six respondents (21%) reported a common survival orientation. A single respondent (3%) reported behavior control as the aim.

Professional Involvement and Group Methods

Helping professionals were frequently involved in the self-help groups reported. Twenty-three of the 29 respondents with groups (79%) reported that a professional regularly attends the group meetings, 5 respondents (17.2%) indicated no professionals attend the self-help group meetings, and 1 respondent (3%) indicated the professional withdrew from the group once it had developed. The role of professionals involved with these groups varied considerably. Respondents were asked to describe the various roles of the professionals meeting with their groups by checking one or more of the following categories: researcher; consultant; trainer; initiator; evaluator; referral agent; and, group leader. Nineteen of the 29 respondents (66%) reported the professional served as a consultant, providing back-up and support to group leaders; 13 respondents (45%) indicated the professional acts as a referral agent, referring patients to self-help groups or other needed services; and, 10 respondents (34%) classified the professional role as that of trainer, offering training in leadership, organizational and group process skills for group members. Ten other respondents (34%) viewed their professional role as a catalyst/initiator, helping to start and organize self-help groups and 7 respondents (24%) reported the professional role as an evaluative one, concerned with assessing the effectiveness of self-help groups. None described the professional role as that of researcher, investigating group dynamics.

One of the issues that has been raised about professional involvement in self-help groups relates to who controls the group. There is potential for conflict between self-help and professional methods of helping; and, if the professional assumes control of a self-help group, the group is less likely to serve as a vehicle for empowerment. In order to determine the possibility of conflict between professionals and members of self-help groups, respondents were asked to assess the extent to which self-help group methods conflict with professional methods of helping by checking one of the following categories: no conflict; very little conflict; moderate conflict; great deal of conflict, or extreme conflict. Seventeen of the 20 respondents (59%) reported no conflict; eight (28%) reported very little conflict; one (3%) reported a great deal of conflict. There were no reports of extreme conflict. Thus, the perceptions of the respondents tend to support the idea that professional involvement is compatible with self-help groups.

Membership and Meeting Arrangements

In order to determine who belonged to these groups, respondents were asked whether patients, family members, or significant others could attend. All of the 29 respondents (100%) indicated patients belonged to the groups. Two respondents (7%) reported groups included parents and patients; the remaining 27 respondents (93%) indicated groups were composed primarily of patients, but others also attended. Eighteen of these respondents (62%) reported that groups were mixed with both family members and significant others attending in addition to patients; the remainder reported that either family members or significant others attended in addition to patients.

Most of the self-help groups reported meeting regularly and holding their meetings in some organizational context in the community. Groups varied in how often and where they met. Fourteen respondents (48%) reported groups meeting monthly; three respondents (10%) reported weekly meetings; two respondents (7%) reported bi-weekly meetings; another two respondents (7%) reported groups meeting periodically, and one respondent (3%) reported on a group that did not meet at all. Further, respondents reported that meetings were held at the following sites: 9 (31%) groups met at a sickle cell clinic, 8 (28%) at an agency-office, 3 (10%) at the homes of patients, 2 (7%) at a hospital, and 1 (3%) at a senior citizen center.

Nature of the Organization

Study respondents were asked to describe the nature of organizational support and affiliation for the self-help groups. Most self-help groups were affiliated with non-profit organizations and made available to patients and families for no fee. Twenty respondents (70%) noted that the identified self-help group was associated with a non-profit organization (two of these were state-affiliated organizations) while 16 (30%) were for profit. Twenty-six respondents (90%) reported on self-help groups that charged no fees. Three respondents (10%) indicated members were charged a fee; and, one of these respondents reported the fee was $1.00 per meeting.

Group Goals

Respondents were asked to consider a list of goals served by self-help groups. All respondents checked more than one goal. Twenty-eight respondents (97%) indicated these groups can be used to help others, to build self-confidence, to meet others with similar problems. Twenty-five (83%) respondents reported that self-help groups offer a sense of empowerment to affect change. Twenty-three respondents (79%) noted that the goals of self-help groups can include gaining a sense of community, dealing with public attitudes and receiving important factual information. Nineteen respondents (66%) checked learning coping skills and strategies, receiving help from others and conveying hope. Answers to an open-ended question about group goals indicated that groups were also used to expand opportunities for individual self-actualization, to raise funds, to improve interpersonal skills, to improve public awareness, to increase patient advocacy, and to develop opportunities for education, training and job placement. Thus, respondents view self-help groups for sickle cell patients and their families as having the capacity to serve multiple goals and offering the opportunity to effect change.

Services Provided

The respondents were asked to describe the type of services provided by sickle cell self-help groups to group members. These services, ranked in order of the frequency with which they were mentioned, include: education (including nutrition counseling), referral services, testing, social events and other activities to reduce isolation, space for meeting, monetary support, psychosocial support, outpatient clinic care, hemoglobin screening services, community education, social casework services, laboratory services, home repair services, interactional and socialization opportunities, job placement services, library resources, job training services, follow-up and supportive services. Thus, these self-help groups provided multiple services.

DISCUSSION

The self-help group movement has gained acceptance with sickle cell patients, families and health care providers. This is evidenced by the large number of respondents reporting the existence of sickle cell groups. The sickle cell staff responding to the survey perceived sickle cell self-help groups as viable vehicles for support, education, proactive networking for patients and providers, and the empowerment of this population.

The data indicate that the majority of the groups identified are ongoing groups, meeting at regularly established times. Respondents considered these groups as valuable resources, capable of enhancing patient effectiveness in personal growth and living. Such groups appear less likely to deal with survival issues related to housing, food, and transportation and are more likely to focus members on enriching considerations, such as education, the service most frequently provided by these groups.

Conflict between the professional role and the self-help group model is reported as minimal. The role of the professional is perceived as a more facilitative and consultative one. This model, as opposed to the clinical therapeutic model where the social worker assumes leadership, is more acceptable to the consumer and is best able to promote the achievement of stated group goals. Patients are responsible for leadership and control in most of the groups. Organizations can support the development of self-help groups by providing a place to meet, mailing and telephone service, and providing professional consultants to sickle cell self-help groups.

Common goals appear to be the basis for the acceptability of these groups to patients and, thus, their apparent success. These include education, support, advocacy, interpersonal skills, technical skills, and activity in the interest of self and community. The common theme of these goals relates to the process of empowerment. This is supported by the number of respondents (25 or 86%) who agreed that self-help groups gave a sense of empowerment to effect change.

This study provides a profile of the self-help groups that have been formed by sickle cell patients and their families. The data, however, raises a number of questions which need to be addressed. Although health benefits to the consumer were noted by the respondents, the specific relationship of self-help groups to improved health status and/or changes in health behavior of sickle cell patients remains unclear. It would be useful to know whether or not individuals who participate in sickle cell self-help groups engage in more positive health behaviors, such as increased compliance with medical regimens, or increased utilization of psychosocial resources or preventive medical practices. Since so many of the groups provide educational services, it would also be important to study the impact of education. Does participation increase knowledge about Sickle Cell Disease and promote a more positive attitude about coping with the disease? Further, the specific knowledge gained and the specific attitudes affected as a result of group participation need to be identified.

Additional research is needed to determine what brings some sickle cell patients to self-help groups and deters others from participating. Research on the characteristics of successful groups would provide further insight into variations in group structure and process, such as frequency of meetings, services provided and level of professional support. Distinctive features of Sickle Cell Disease, such as its chronicity and its primary impact on Blacks, magnify the importance of the emergence of self-help groups and self-help activities as a vehicle for empowerment.

The sickle cell self-help movement, documented by this survey, supports the concept of helping to empower this patient population. When self-help groups are available as an addition to the existing delivery system, sickle cell patients and their families have the opportunity to develop competencies that enhance their sense of self-worth, to pursue personal interests, and to make changes in their environment. The data gathered from these 29 respondents provide a clearer sense of the goals, membership patterns, frequency of meetings, relationships with professionals, and services rendered by self-help groups that are available for sickle cell patients and their families. The flexibility of self-help groups as a mechanism for empowerment is demonstrated by the varied membership and multiple goals. The support, education, counseling, advocacy, networking, and mutual exchange offered by these groups have the potential for empowering members so they can function more effectively.

REFERENCES

Alleyne, S.I., Wint, E., & Serjeant, G.R. (1976). Psychosocial aspects of sickle cell disease. *Health and Social Work, 1*(4), 1-7.

Antonousky, A. (1980). *Health, stress, and coping.* San Francisco: Jossey-Bass.

Battle, S. (1984). Sickle cell anemia: Implications for genetic counseling in social work practice. *Pediatric Social Work, 2*(4), 111-117.

Black, R.B. & Drachman, D. (1985). Hospital social workers and self-help groups. *Health and Social Work, 10*(2), 95-105.

Bowman, J.E. (1983). Identification and stigma in the workplace. In J.O. Weiss, B.A. Bernhardt, & N.W. Paul (Eds.), *Genetic disorders and birth defects in families and society: Toward interdisciplinary understanding.* (pp. 223-229). White Plains, NY: March of Dimes Birth Defects Foundation.

Briscoe, G. (1986). *The psychosocial impact of sickle cell anemia: A review.* Unpublished manuscript. University of Cincinnati Comprehensive Sickle Cell Center.

Chamberlain, N., Nash, K.B., & Woodward, K.W. (1973-1974). Indications of stress in families with sickle cell anemia members and the relationship to health care delivery. In H.L. Olson & N. Dahl (Eds.), *Inventory of marriage and family literature.* (Vol. III, pp. 377-394). Minneapolis, MN: University of Minneapolis Press.

Chesler, M. & Barbarin, O. (1986). *Childhood cancer and family.* New York: Brunner-Mansel.

Chesler, M. & Chesney O. (1988). Self-help groups: Empowerment and behaviors of disabled and chronically ill persons. In H.E. Yuker (Ed.), *Attitudes toward persons with disabilities.* (pp. 230-247). New York: Springer Publishing Company.

Conyard, W., Krishnamurthy, M., & Dosile, H. (1980). Psychosocial aspects of sickle cell anemia in adolescents. *Health and Social Work, 5,* 20-25.

Corley, P. (1986, April). *Factors affecting participation levels.* Paper presented at the National Conference, Sickle Cell Disease: Progress and Prospects, Boston, MA.

Evans, C.F. (1983, November). *Self-help groups: Fortifying the potential.* Paper presented at the National Conference, Sickle Cell Disease: Research and Social Scientific Perspectives, Chicago, IL.

Evans, C.F. (1985, March). Self-help groups: The patient's perspective. Paper presented at the National Conference, Sickle Cell Disease, Los Angeles, CA.

Evans, R.C., Burlew, A.K., & Oler, C.H. (1988). Children with sickle cell anemia: Parental relations, parent-child relations, and child behavior. *Social Work,* 127-130.

Featherstone, H. (1980). *A difference in the family.* New York: Basic Books.

Johnson, C. (1981). Sickle cell disease. In W. Stolov & M. Clowers (Eds.), *Handbook of severe disability.* (pp. 349-362). Washington, DC: U.S. Department of Education.

Katz, A. (1980). Toward understanding of self-help groups. *High Hopes, A Forum for Perinatal Social Workers, 3,* 1-12.

Katz, A. (1984). What self-help groups can contribute to genetic disorders. *Proceedings of the National Conference on Self-Help Groups for Genetic Disorders.* (pp. 7-22). Washington, DC.

Lurie, A. & Schulman, L. (1983). The professional connection with self-help groups in health care settings. *Social Work in Health Care, 8,* 69-70.

Motulsky, A.G. (1973). Frequency of sickling disorder in U.S. blacks. *New England Journal of Medicine, 222,* 31-33.

Nash, K.B. (1983). Overview of humanistic progress in sickle cell anemia during the past ten years. *The American Journal of Pediatric Hematology/Oncology*, 5(4), 352-359.

Nash, K.B. (1986). Ethnicity, race, and health care delivery system as it pertains to sickle cell anemia. In A. Hurtig & C.T. Viera (Eds.), *Sickle cell disease: Psychological and psychosocial issues*. (pp. 131-146). Champagne: University of Illinois Press.

Nishiura, E., Whitten, C.F., & Jenkins, D. (1980, August). Screening for psychosocial problems in health settings. *Health and Social Work*, 5(3), 22-28.

Paz, J. (1984). *Empowerment: Strengthening the natural support network of the hispanic rural elder*. Unpublished manuscript, Howard University, Washington, DC.

Scott, R.B. (1979). Reflections on the current status of the sickle cell disease program in the United States. *Journal of National Medical Association*, 71, 679-681.

Smith, J.A. (1983). Management of sickle cell disease: Progress during the past ten years. *The American Journal of Pediatric Hematology/Oncology*, 5(4), 360-366.

Solomon, B. (1976). *Black empowerment: Social work in oppressed communities*. (pp. 11-30). New York: Columbia University Press.

Taylor, S. (1979). Hospital patient behavior: Reactions, helplessness, or control. *Journal of Social Services*, 3-5(1), 156-184.

Toseland, R.W. & Hacker, L. (1982). Self-help groups and professional involvement. *Social Work*, 27, 341-347.

Vavasseur, J. (1977). A comprehensive program for meeting psychological needs of sickle cell anemia patients. *Journal of National Medical Association*, 69, 335.

Whitten, C.F. (1982). A decade of sickle cell awareness, progress, and challenges. *Urban Health*, 11, 43.

Whitten, C. & Fischoff, J. (1974). Psychological effects of sickle cell disease. *Archives of Internal Medicine*, 33, 681-689.

Williams, I., Earles, A., & Pack, B. (1983). Psychological considerations in sickle cell disease. *Nurse Clinics of North America*, 18, 215-229.

Coping with a First Heart Attack: A Group Treatment Model for Low-Income Anglo, Black, and Hispanic Patients

Karen Subramanian
Kathleen O. Ell

SUMMARY. The stressful effects of both poverty and racism contribute to the fact that heart disease is a leading cause of death for poor and minority populations. In spite of this, there is an absence of reported psychosocial interventions with these vulnerable populations. This paper describes a structured group treatment model based on cognitive-behavioral interventions for lower SES Anglo, Black, and Hispanic patients who have had a heart attack. The rationale for using this approach is developed through a review of the literature, and the treatment strategy is described in some detail.

Epidemiological data continue to document higher coronary heart disease morbidity and mortality rates among the poor and minority groups (Marmot, Adelstein, Robinson, & Rose, 1978; Morgenstern, 1980; Rene, 1987). Indeed, there is evidence that Blacks (Rene, 1987) and the poor have been slower to experience the overall population decline in ischemic heart disease mortality (Wing, Casper, Riggan et al., 1988). It is likely, therefore, that many social workers in health care serve substantial numbers of poor and minority patients who have experienced a life-threatening cardiac event.

Karen Subramanian, PhD, and Kathleen O. Ell, DSW, are affiliated with the School of Social Work, University of Southern California.

This program was funded in part by the Faculty Research and Innovation Fund of the University of Southern California.

Unfortunately, the literature on psychosocial interventions for such patients is exceedingly sparse.

In a beginning attempt to address this gap on the practice literature, this paper presents a coping skills group model designed for lower socioeconomic (SES) Anglo, Black and Hispanic patients recovering from a first heart attack (myocardial infarction). This group model is designed to enhance patients' adaptation to a first heart attack by enhancing their sense of control, social support, and coping repertoires. The rationale for the use of cognitive-behavioral strategies is presented followed by a detailed description of the group model.

The goals of the group model are based on a previously reported longitudinal study of post-myocardial infarction (MI) recovery among different sociocultural groups (Ell & Haywood, 1985; 1985-86). In that study, a patient's personal sense of control and social support were found to be important predictors of that patient's subsequent psychological and functional adaptation. Most important, significant differences in anxiety, functional status, and self-reported health status were found among lower SES Blacks, Hispanics, and Anglos when compared with upper SES Anglos. In addition, there were significant differences in personal sense of control, beliefs about recovery, coping responses, and social support systems between these two SES populations. Other recent studies of coping with serious illness support several of these study results (Ell, 1985-86; Ell, Nishimoto, Mantell, & Hamovitch, in press; Ell, Nishimoto, Morvay, Mantell, & Hamovitch, in press), emphasizing the need to design psychosocial interventions to address patients' personal and social coping resources.

The importance of social support in recovery from a MI is well-documented (Ell & Dunkel-Schetter, in press; Waltz, 1986a, 1986b). At the same time, unhelpful primary network support has been shown to cancel out helpful support (Ell & Haywood, 1985). For example, evidence suggests that family conflict is common during hospitalization and early convalescence (Ell & Dunkel-Schetter, in press). This conflict is frequently centered on patient activity levels and is exacerbated when patients and family members receive inadequate information from health care professionals or when the information is poorly understood. Furthermore, in the study of MI recovery, lower SES Anglo patients reported a significant decline in social support from intimate network members over time, whereas the other groups reported no such decline (Ell & Haywood, 1985-86). This finding was especially disturbing in view of the fact that support had the greatest influence on adaptation for lower SES Anglos. Interventions are needed, therefore, to assist patients in their ability to obtain both informational and emotional support and to sustain access to support after the acute phase of illness.

The need for the development and assessment of specific models of treatment for minority populations has been highlighted by Jones (1985) who stresses that the recent proliferation of literature on cross-cultural counseling and psychotherapy, while being an important advance, is at a level of generality that is inadequate for the therapist who is ready to begin a treatment program. The recent literature on working with lower SES minorities has refuted the earlier belief that this population could not benefit from treatment (Acosta & Evans, 1982; Bass, Acosta, & Evans, 1982; Herrera & Sanchez, 1976).

COGNITIVE-BEHAVIORAL THERAPY

A review of the cognitive-behavioral literature indicates that this theoretical approach can be congruent with the needs and expectations of lower SES Anglo, Black, and Hispanic heart patients. In the cognitive-behavioral approach, the clients' problems are believed to be caused by a combination of skill or learning deficits, lack of positive sanctions or reinforcements, illogical or self-depreciating thought patterns, and physical reactions to high levels of stress. An educational climate is fostered and interventions are usually active, time-limited, and structured. Thus, the focus is on learning coping skills to help manage current problems and stresses (Kendall & Hollon, 1979). The approach includes a climate which promotes the value of patient self-control, collaboration with the clinician, and self-help responsibility.

Studies indicate that cardiac patients want assistance in getting well physically, solving immediate problems, and planning for future tasks. These patients want to know the facts of their illness, do not wish to be introspective, and are not responsive to traditional insight-oriented groups (Hackett, 1978). The cognitive-behavioral approach emphasizes the patient as learner in an educationally-focused model. Research indicates that the most useful counseling for cardiac patients seems to be fairly specific and educational, although the presence of group support may enhance the effect (Blanchard & Miller, 1977; Rahe, Ward, & Hayes, 1979). Studies also indicate that education can decrease the frequency with which patients experience anxiety, depression, treatment problems, dissatisfaction related to work performance, and unhappiness related to personal appearance and sexual intimacy.

Several investigators have advocated that the treatment of lower SES clients should attempt to employ a problem-oriented approach focusing both on present circumstances and design of active interventions as opposed to the traditional modalities emphasizing interpersonal dynamics and insight (Garfield, 1971; Cohen, 1972; Normand, Iglesias, & Payn, 1974; Reissman & Scheibner, 1965). Smith and Dejoie-Smith (1984) claim that behavior therapy is more appropriate for or more likely to be "effective" (in terms of attrition rate, subjective client satisfaction, client receptivity, or client improvement) with non-white and lower SES clients. In their view, the effectiveness of behavior therapy for this population is due to the immediate and direct response to clients' problems; the use of methods (directive, concrete, reinforcing) that more closely conform to the life experiences and expectations of poor and minority clients; and the focus on observable behaviors which offer less room for "victim blaming" or biased interpretations.

Cognitive-behavioral therapy recognizes cultural differences in its assessment and intervention strategies (Jenkins, Rahaim, Kelly, & Payne, 1982; Higginbothan & Tanaka-Matsumi, 1981). The self-help orientation of the therapy can be of benefit in reducing the role of prejudice since the emphasis on becoming self-sufficient eliminates the client's "one-down" role in treatment (Jones, 1985; Maultsby, 1982) and dependency on the therapist. Some authors believe that the cognitive-behavioral assessment model which stresses the individual as a learner and measures increasing competence in various areas rather than personality changes can remove many forms of resistance to service and enhance cooperation with disadvantaged populations (Garvin, 1985; Smith & Dejoie-Smith,

1984). There is evidence that the cognitive-behavioral approach is effective in helping Hispanic men and women resolve problems of depression and family conflicts (Arce & Torres-Matrullo, 1982) as well as help Black clients cope with life stressors (Groves, 1982; Turner, & Jones, 1982).

Assertiveness is the behavioral skill most frequently mentioned as beneficial to lower SES and minority clients. Given that lower SES cardiac patients are less knowledgeable about the illness and more reluctant to actively seek information, changing client behaviors so that clients will communicate on their own behalf is a desired goal of treatment (Acosta, Yamamoto, Evans, & Wilcox, 1982; Garvin, 1985). It is important to note, however, that there is a paucity of empirical data demonstrating cognitive-behavioral therapy's greater effectiveness with lower SES and minority clients. Just as with any other type of psychotherapy, the effectiveness of cognitive-behavioral therapy is affected by the therapist's sensitivity to culture, race, or ethical issues.

THE PROPOSED TREATMENT MODEL

Use of the Group Format

The use of groups in the health field is widespread and the benefits of the approach are frequently reported in the practice literature (Carlton, 1984; Lonergan, 1982; Perry, 1980). There is, however, little documentation of group work with lower SES and minority patients, although the few reports available indicate that group work can be an effective means of serving this population (Davis, 1984; Garvin, 1985; Herrera & Sanchez, 1976). For example, groups which provide an opportunity for mutual aid and role-modeling to enhance members' abilities to cope with reformulation of their personal roles and coping strategies is effective among lower SES Black and Hispanic patients with hypertension (Maida, 1985). Skill groups in particular can help oppressed clients become more effective in communications and networking (Garvin, 1985), skills that are important in dealing with one's family, friends, community resources, and health care providers.

The group method has been reported to be helpful to cardiac patients (Hackett, 1978; Hackett & Cassem, 1982). Depression is considered to be one of the most formidable problems in cardiac convalescence and rehabilitation (Ell & Dunkel-Schetter, in press), yet the very act of coming to a group counters the routine passivity of being ill (Lonergan, 1982). Group settings promote patients interacting with and helping each other, thus offsetting the possible loss of social interaction within their normal social environment. Information presented which stimulates various questions and situations from group members can also help to alleviate depression caused by fears and myths.

It has been frequently recommended in the literature that group treatment for lower SES and minority patients be time-limited and action-oriented (Acosta & Yamamoto, 1984; Garvin, 1985; Lorion, 1978). This format is also preferred by cardiac patients in general (Hackett, 1978). With continually rising health care costs, financing long-term psychosocial intervention for patients is increasingly impractical and those therapies designed for specific and limited time intervals meet the need to consider economic considerations.

Goals and Strategies of the Treatment Group

The goals of the group treatment include the provision of information about illness and cardiac recovery, community resources, and the management of illness and non-illness related stressors, including family relationships in daily living. Goals also include increasing patients' coping skills in order to improve their ability to mobilize personal and formal support systems and manage stress.

Group treatment strategies are primarily educational, involving mini-lectures and discussions, and the teaching of problem-solving skills. Training in problem-solving can increase a patient's sense of control by enhancing perceptions of competence and self-efficacy in dealing with new events and problems, and can help patients gain resources and mobilize support systems. Assertiveness training can be taught within a problem-solving model using behavioral rehearsal, a simulation of the client's actual or anticipated behavior in a troublesome situation (Wells, 1982). The social skills deficiencies of lower SES and minority individuals have been found to be amenable to change using this method (Boulettte, 1976; Herrera & Sanchez, 1976; Maida, 1985). Behavioral rehearsal becomes a format for practicing problem-solving skills in that it includes definition of the problem, brainstorming to generate possible solutions, selection and evaluation of each alternative, implementation, and evaluation of the effort (Rose, 1984).

Behavioral rehearsals which practice problem-solving might involve stressors related to the health care system, family life, or formal support systems. Learning to ask physicians and other health care personnel questions about medication or changes in life style is essential to good recovery. In order to gain correct medical information, patients must formulate their question, practice asking in an assertive manner, develop and practice follow-up questions, and be able to check-out their understanding of the information received. Family issues to be rehearsed might include requesting a spouse to be less overprotective or asking help from an estranged son or daughter. Even a simple call to the local American Heart Association or to the Social Security office can become an obstacle if patients do not have the confidence that skills training can develop.

Cognitive skills will be introduced only briefly to patients due to the time constraints of treatment and the fact that there is less evidence to indicate the effectiveness of these skills with the target population. Cognitive skills will focus on constructive thinking as related to feelings management. Common dysfunctional thinking patterns might include "Life is over for me," "I'll never recover," and "If I can't be the way I was before, I'm no good anymore." Patients will first become aware of the relationship of thinking to feelings and behavior when an early group discussion of myths about heart attacks is demonstrated to affect patients' affect and behavior. For example, the belief that any exercise may bring on a heart attack can lead to continual anxiety about mobility which may be demonstrated in angry verbal attacks on family members. Later in the group, this sequence of thinking, feeling, and behaving will be generalized to other beliefs of the patients.

Suggestions for the empirical evaluation of the group include the initial use of single case design because of the small number of subjects in each group (Jayaratne, 1978). After a number of groups have been completed, additional information can be gained by combining the pre and post data for all subjects, providing a group rather than individual result. The goals of this treatment model can be operationalized with respect to measures of social support, locus of control, and stress levels. Several resources for selecting assessment instruments are available for the practitioner (Corcoran & Fischer, 1987; Hudson, 1982). Because of potential literacy problems with this population, all assessment measures should be interviewer-administered.

Number and Sequence of Group Sessions

The model presented includes a combination of 2 inpatient and 2 outpatient group sessions. The inpatient group sessions should be scheduled for 1 hour each the last two days the patient is in the hospital. Limiting the number of hospital sessions to 2 meetings recognizes the current realities of shorter hospital stays, the fatigue of the patient, and the need for the patient to be available for medical procedures. The remaining 2 sessions, 1 1/2 hours in length, should be completed during the patient's first two follow-up visits. It is expected that the average length of time between these follow-up visits will be 4-6 weeks. Coordination between the group leader and physician is essential so that members of a particular group can be scheduled for their follow-up visits on the same days.

The group leader should remind patients about the group meeting on the day of the group as their illness and hospital procedures may be uppermost on their minds. Patients should be called twice between each outpatient session, once midway between sessions and once a few days before the session begins. This is essential not only to motivate and encourage patients to return to the group, but to make sure that they can still be contacted at a previous address or phone number. Patients who do not have phones can be sent reminder letters, but it is best to attempt to reach a friend or relative who can verbally remind the patient.

Pre-Group Preparation and Recruitment

In planning an intervention strategy for poor and ethnic minority patients, the practitioner is faced with two general tasks. First, the practitioner must gain knowledge of the varied cultural norms and develop skills in working with the patients. Successful completion of this task prepares the practitioner to adapt techniques, especially the level of activity; the ability to communicate acceptance and respect for the client in terms that are culturally specific, intelligible, and meaningful; and to be open to the need for direct intervention in the life circumstances of the patient (Draguns, 1981). Second, practitioners are challenged never to lose sight of the fact that there is a substantial variation within sub-population groups. Practitioners are reminded to routinely assess patients' ethnic self-identity, language, religion, family ties, and acculturation levels to ensure that knowledge of cultural group differences does not obscure the unique individuality of a particular patient (Jones, 1985).

Anglo, Black, and Hispanic lower SES patients who have had a first heart attack can be referred to the group leader by the ward nurse or staff social worker. Social workers assigned to cardiac units may take both roles. Nurses are valuable allies in group recruitment not only because they see the patients on a daily basis, but also because they know and can identify the doctors who need to be solicited for permission for group attendance. Further, nurses have important knowledge about hospital procedures and can suggest a time for the group to meet when members will not be interrupted by normal hospital routine. As soon as patients have been released from intensive care, they can be identified and physician permission obtained. This will allow sufficient time for procedures before the group actually begins.

When the group includes Hispanic patients, both the initial contact person and one of the group leaders must have fluency in Spanish, and Hispanic patients should be asked (when it is not obvious) whether they would prefer an English or Spanish-speaking group. Although it has been repeatedly indicated that fluency in a particular language is essential for a successful group (Maida, 1985; Padilla & Salgado De Snyder, 1985), other types of heterogeneity (such as race, ethnicity, sex, or age) are well tolerated by patients in medical crisis situations (Longergan, 1982; Maida, 1985). Because of the short-term nature of treatment, limiting the group to 5-6 patients will allow more group time for members to practice the skills. More members should be included when attrition due to transportation problems, illness, or reluctance to attend appear likely once patients leave the hospital.

Socialization to group treatment begins when the group leader meets and talks with patients individually to invite them to the group. The use of preparation techniques is a valuable treatment adjunct for lower SES and minority clients whose pre-therapy expectations often differ from those of their therapists and who may not have known other individuals who have gone through the therapeutic process and could serve as models (Cobb, 1972; Heitler, 1973; Heitler, 1976). Pre-intervention in the form of information about the nature and process of therapy assists the client in understanding how best to participate in therapy. The client may then be more self-disclosing and willing to express feelings, needs, and expectations of therapy in such a way that the benefits of counseling are maximized (Bass, Acosta, & Evans, 1982; Mayo, 1974).

For example, it may be particularly important to explain the value of therapy to Hispanic patients because their cultures stress the concept that men must be strong and stoic, and the open discussion of personal problems may be viewed as a sign of weakness or inferiority (Herrera & Sanchez, 1976; Schreiber & Homiak, 1981). For Black patients, the educational focus of the group should be emphasized since the beginning phase of a racially heterogeneous treatment group may be very anxiety arousing and lack of trust may be an issue that deters involvement (Davis, 1984). The educational focus can be viewed as less threatening than an insight-oriented group as it requires less cohesiveness, trust, self-disclosure, and focus on personality change.

Description of Sessions

Session 1

The goals for the first group meeting in the hospital include:

1. To provide an overall rationale for treatment and a connection to members' own beliefs about health and illness;
2. To present information about the causes of heart attacks and to elicit and correct myths about the illness;
3. To allow for beginning self-disclosure and development of group cohesiveness.

The first session begins with an exercise that allows group members to meet one another and discover their commonalities in order to begin the basis of social support and social comparison that the group will provide. This can be done either by going around the room or using other exercises that allow members to introduce one another. Based on evidence that Hispanics appreciate knowing their group leader as a person and that trust may initially be lacking for Blacks, the leader should be sure to provide a short introduction in order to establish his/her humanity as well as professional credentials. In order to encourage expression of feelings and make clear commonalities among members, a short case study about a patient similar to the group members can be described by the leader. Then the leader would facilitate a discussion of members' similarities and differences to that patient. As patients are able to share their concerns freely, cohesiveness among members will develop, allowing members to eventually increase their participation.

Information about the members' illness can be presented in short mini-lecture form (10 minutes) with discussion following. The use of pictures or short films is encouraged as a way to catch and maintain the patients' interest. Information on the etiology of heart disease to be presented includes personal attributes such as age, sex, race, and heredity, as well as behavioral factors such as diet and smoking. Popular myths and misperceptions about life after a heart attack should be clarified. Common myths that heart patients believe include the dangers of all forms of exercise, a second heart attack taking place on the anniversary of the first one, and issues surrounding sexuality. Educational literature is available in both Spanish and English from the American Heart Association and can be distributed in the group, having a secondary benefit of acquainting group members with this agency as a resource.

The presentation of information should not be a one-way process. As medical information about the illness, medications, and acceptable activity levels is presented, the patients' fears and cultural beliefs about these subjects should be solicited for discussion purposes. Cultural beliefs that differ from scientific information should be regarded as alternative systems and not "wrong." Unless they are discussed, however, patients may not be able to accept the new information that they are being presented.

Session 2

The goals for the second group meeting in the hospital include:

1. To introduce the relationship of stress to illness and recovery;
2. To elicit the members' most immediate sources of stress;
3. To present and practice problem-solving through behavioral rehearsal.

Since stress is an important issue in illness and recovery, a short mini-lecture with visual aids and discussion about stressors and physical reactions to these stressors in the lives of the members can educate as well as raise awareness of this issue. It is possible that a few members will not be able to read or write. Thus, it may be useful for the worker to use pictures taped to a board as a means of listing the stressors. Discussion should also involve ways in which members physically notice the onset of stress.

The list of stressors developed by members will probably include issues of daily living such as family, self-image, friends, and how to change diet and smoking behaviors. Psychological concerns such as depression and anxiety and bodily concerns involving confusion about the interpretation and proper remedial action for chest pains are both common area of stress. The patients will also want to discuss work, finances, and social service resources because lower SES patients will frequently experience work-related and financial problems of a more serious nature than middle- and upper-class patients. It is essential, therefore, that the social worker have knowledge of community social resources in order to present this to patients.

In addition to the presentation of information, work on the priority list of stressors is approached through a problem-solving behavioral rehearsal format. The group worker can guide each patient through the problem-solving method, asking for discussion and suggestions from group members when appropriate. Role-playing with the leader as well as other groups members will clarify possible obstacles to resolving the problem. The behavioral rehearsal format will be important for patients as they discuss restructuring family relationships as well as utilizing social resources. Even patients with knowledge of social agencies may need practice in the group to be able to obtain what they need from these resources. Role-play practice in making telephone calls, how to ask questions of medical personnel, etc., will ensure implementation more than would just the presentation of information.

By the end of the second session, the group worker will have some knowledge about the social needs of each member and may find it beneficial to make initial calls to social resources on behalf of some of the group members. Although the ultimate goal of the treatment is to empower patients to become more effective at obtaining resources for themselves, it is also true that oppressed people at times need direct intervention from the social worker to gain information and resources. This becomes an even more important issue when one is working with a very ill individual.

Session 3

The goals for this third group meeting, which is the first outpatient session, include:

1. To review material presented in first 2 sessions;
2. To establish a priority list of patients' current sources of stress;
3. To problem solve through behavioral rehearsal.

There will be a necessary re-orientation to group goals and group members in this first outpatient session. One way to accomplish this task while encouraging group participation and assessing how much was retained from the inpatient sessions is to have group members lead this discussion, with the group leader intervening as necessary. As in Session 2, the leader will become aware of certain issues that may require social work intervention — in particular, issues related to obtaining help from formal support systems. The ideal way to approach these issues would be in cooperation with the patient; the patient completing a task discussed and practiced in the group, and the leader doing follow-up to enhance the chances of success. For example, the patient can rehearse a telephone call to the hospital to find out when a clinic visit will be scheduled. If this call is assigned as "homework," the social worker can then contact the patient to determine whether the information was successfully obtained. If not, the social worker can make further suggestions or assist personally in obtaining the information.

The problem-solving behavioral rehearsal format introduced in Session 2 will be continued here as further disclosure continues of patients' personal problems and social needs that they have experienced in their 4 to 6 weeks out of the hospital. Although group members may need to be reminded about the problem-solving and behavioral rehearsal methods used in Session 2, their prior use of these methods should result in more effective problem-solving. The choice of stressors to be discussed should be made by the group as a whole and will probably be divided between financial, family, and health concerns.

Session 4

The goals for the last outpatient session include:

1. To continue problem-solving through behavioral rehearsal;
2. To discuss constructive thoughts and their relation to feelings management.

The first part of this session will be very similar to Session 3. By the fourth session, however, patients may be more willing to express their thoughts and fears about the illness and concerns about coping with the problems of recovery; thus, the second half of the session should introduce the concept of constructive thoughts. Concerns about death and dying, feelings of depression, guilt about non-performance of former social roles, etc., may be issues for the patients. As thoughts about these issues are brought forth in the group, the leader can then label them as constructive (realistic, leading towards coping and feeling good about yourself) or non-constructive (not realistic, leading towards apathy, inaction, and negative feelings) and reinforce the former. Emphasis will be placed on helping patients discover their strengths for coping that they may not have recognized before.

CONCLUSION

This treatment model is based on the premise that lower SES and minority individuals have higher illness and mortality rates and are at a disadvantage in coping with illness-related stress. Despite this need, few treatment programs have been developed to serve this population. The proposed model suggests specific ways in which known approaches can be targeted for these vulnerable individuals.

Although this is a very short treatment program, the authors believe that it is worth developing and evaluating based on the evidence that many of these patients attempting to cope with a first heart attack receive little or no psychosocial treatment. It is hoped that as a result of such treatments, patients will experience lower levels of stress, enhance their personal and social support networks, reclaim some measure of personal control, learn problem-solving skills, and experience a less problematic illness course and optimal adaptation.

REFERENCES

Acosta, F.X. & Evans, A. (1982). The Hispanic American patient. In F.X. Acosta, J. Yamamoto & A. Evans (Eds.), *Effective psychotherapy for low income minority patients* (pp. 51-82). New York: Plenum Press.

Acosta, F.X. & Yamamoto, J. (1984). The utility of group work practice for Hispanic Americans. *Social Work with Groups, 7,* 63-73.

Acosta, F.X., Yamamoto, J. & Evans, A. (1982). *Effective psychotherapy for low income minority patients.* New York: Plenum Press.

Arce, A. & Torres-Matrullo, C. (1982). Application of cognitive behavioral techniques in the treatment of Hispanic patients. *Psychiatric Quarterly, 54,* 230-236.

Bandura, A. (1982). Self-efficacy mechanism in human agency. *American Psychologist, 37,* 122-147.

Bass, B.A., Acosta, F.X. & Evans, A. (1982). The Black American patient. In F.X. Acosta, J. Yamamoto & A. Evans (Eds.), *Effective psychotherapy for low income minority patients* (pp. 83-108). New York: Plenum Press.

Blanchard, E.B. & Miller, S.T. (1977). Psychological treatment of cardiovascular disease. *Archives of General Psychiatry, 34,* 1402-1413.

Boulette, T.R. (1976). Assertive training with low income Mexican American Women. In M.R. Miranda (Ed.), *Psychotherapy with the Spanish-Speaking: Issues in research and service delivery* (pp. 67-72). Los Angeles: Spanish Speaking Mental Health Research Center.

114   GROUPS IN HEALTH CARE SETTINGS

Carlton, T.O. (1984). *Clinical social work in health settings*. New York: Springer Publishing Co.

Cassem, N.H. & Hackett, T.P. (1971). Psychiatric consultation in a coronary care unit. *Annals of Internal Medicine, 75*, 9-14.

Cobb, C. (1972). Community mental health services and the lower socioeconomic class: A summary of research literature on outpatient treatment (1963-1969). *American Journal of Orthopsychiatry, 42*, 404-414.

Cohen, R. (1972). Principles of preventive mental health programs for ethnic minority populations: The acculturation of Puerto Ricans to the United States. *American Journal of Psychiatry, 128*, 1529-1533.

Corcoran, K. & Fischer, J. (1987). *Measures for clinical practice*. New York: The Free Press.

Croog, S.H. & Levine, S. (1969). Social status and psychological perceptions of 250 men after myocardial infarction. *Health Reports, 84*, 989-993.

Davis, L.E. (1984). Essential components of group work with Black Americans. *Social Work with Groups, 7*, 97-109.

Draguns, J.G. (1981). Counseling across cultures: Common themes and distinct approaches. In P.B. Pedersen, J.G. Draguns, W.J. Lonner & J.E. Trimble (Eds.), *Counseling across cultures* (pp. 3-21). Honolulu: University Press of Hawaii.

Ell, K.O. (1985-86). Coping with serious illness: On integrating constructs to enhance clinical research, assessment and intervention. *International Journal of Psychiatry in Medicine, 15*, 335-355.

Ell, K.O. & Dundel-Schetter, C. (in press). Social support and adjustment to myocardial infarction, angioplasty and coronary artery bypass surgery. In S.A. Shumaker & S.M. Czajkowski (Eds.), *Social support and cardiovascular disease*. New York: Plenum Press.

Ell, K.O., Nishimoto, R., Mantell, J. & Hamovitch, M. (in press). Social support, sense of control and coping among patients with breast, colorectal or lung cancer. *Journal of Psychosocial Oncology*.

Ell, K.O., Nishimoto, R., Morvay, T., Mantell, J. & Hamovitch, M. (in press). A longitudinal analysis of psychological adaptation among survivors of cancer. *Cancer*.

Ell, K.O. & Haywood, L.J. (1985). Clinical implications of patients' sense of control and social support in MI recovery. *Urban Health, 14*, 31-34.

Ell, K.O. & Haywood, L.J. (1985-86). Sociocultural factors in MI recovery: An exploratory study. *International Journal of Psychiatry in Medicine, 15*(2), 157-175.

Garfield, S. (1971). Research on client variables in psychotherapy. In A. Bergin & S. Garfield (Eds.), *Handbook of psychotherapy and behavior change*. New York: John Wiley and Sons.

Garvin, C.D. (1985). Work with disadvantaged and oppressed groups. In M. Sundel, P. Glasser, R. Sarri, & R. Vinter (Eds.), *Individual change through small groups* (pp. 461-472). New York: The Free Press.

Groves, G. (1982). Stress disorders. In S.M. Turner & R.T. Jones (Eds.), *Behavior modification in black populations* (pp. 279-300). New York: Plenum Press.

Hackett, T.P. (1978). The use of groups in the rehabilitation of the postcoronary patient. *Advanced Cardiology, 24,* 127-135.

Hacket, T.P. & Cassem, N.H. (1982). Coping with cardiac disease. *Advanced Cardiology, 31,* 212-217.

Hackett, T.P. & Cassem, N.H. (1976). White-collar and blue-collar responses to heart attack. *Journal of Psychosomatic Research, 20,* 85-95.

Heitler, J.B. (1976). Preparatory techniques in initiating expressive psychotherapy with lower-class, unsophisticated patients. *Psychological Bulletin, 83,* 339-352.

Heitler, J.B. (1973). Preparation of lower-class patients for expressive group psychotherapy. *Journal of Consulting and Clinical Psychology, 41,* 251-260.

Herrera, A.E. & Sanchez, V.C. (1976). Behaviorally oriented group therapy: A successful application in the treatment of low income Spanish-speaking clients. In M.R. Miranda (Ed.), *Psychotherapy with the Spanish-speaking: Issues in research and service delivery* (pp. 73-84). Los Angeles: Spanish Speaking Mental Health Research Center.

Higginbothan, H.N. & Tanaka-Matsumi, J. (1981). Behavioral approaches to counseling across cultures. In P. Pedersen, J. Draguns, W. Lonner & J. Trimble (Eds.), *Counseling across cultures* (pp. 247-274). Hawaii: The University Press.

Hudson, W.W. (1982). *The clinical measurement package.* Homewood, Ill.: The Dorsey Press.

Jayaratne, S. (1978). Analytic procedures for single subject design. *Social Work Research and Abstracts, 14,* 30-40.

Jenkins, J.O., Rahaim, S., Kelly, L.M. & Payne, D. (1982). Substance abuse. In S.M. Turner & R.T. Jones (Eds.), *Behavior modification in Black populations* (pp. 209-248). New York: Plenum Press.

Jones, E.E. (1985). Psychotherapy and counseling with Black clients. In P. Pedersen (Ed.), *Handbook of cross cultural counseling and therapy* (pp. 173-180). Westport, Conn.: Greenwood Press.

Kendall, P.C. & Hollon, S.D. (1979). *Cognitive behavioral interventions.* New York: Academic Press.

Lonergan, E.C. (1982). Discussion of use of groups in the health field. In A. Lurie, G. Rosenberg & S. Pinsky (Eds.), *Social work with groups in health settings.* New York: Prodist.

Lorion, R.P. (1978). Research on psychotherapy and behavior change with the disadvantaged. In S.L. Garfield & A.E. Bergin (Eds.), *Handbook of psychotherapy and behavior change: An empirical analysis* (pp. 903-938). New York: Wiley.

Lorion, R.P. (1973). Socioeconomic status and traditional treatment approaches reconsidered. *Psychological Bulletin, 79,* 263-270.

Maida, Carl A. (1985). Social support and learning in preventive health care. *Social Science in Medicine, 21,* 335-339.

Marmot, M.G., Adelstein, A.M., Robinson, N. & Rose, G.A. (1978). Changing social class distribution of heart disease. *British Medical Journal, 2,* 1109-1112.

Maultsby, M.C., Jr. (1982). A historical view of Blacks' distrust of psychiatry. In S.M. Turner & R.T. Jones (Eds.), *Behavior modification in Black populations* (pp. 151-170). New York: Plenum Press.

Mayo, J.A. (1974). The significance of sociocultural variables in the psychiatric treatment of Black outpatients. *Comprehensive Psychiatry, 15,* 471-482.

Morgenstern, H. (1980). The changing association between social status and coronary heart disease in a rural population. *Social Science and Medicine, 14A,* 191-201.

Normand, W., Iglesias, J. & Payne, S. (1974). Brief group therapy to facilitate utilization of mental health services by Spanish-speaking patients. *American Journal of Orthopsychiatry, 44,* 37-42.

Padilla, A.M. & Salgado De Snyder, N. (1985). Counseling Hispanics: Strategies for effective intervention. In P. Pederson (Ed.), *Handbook of cross-cultural counseling and therapy* (pp. 157-164). Westport, Conn.: Greenwood Press.

Perry, J.K. (1980). Group services for the chronically ill and disabled. *Social Work with Groups, 3,* 59-67.

Perlin, L.D., Lieberman, M.A., Managhan, E.G. & Mullan, J.T. (1986). The stress process. *Journal of Health and Social Behavior, 22,* 337-356.

Rahe, R.H., Ward, H.W. & Hayes, V. (1979). Brief group therapy in myocardial infarction rehabilitation: Three-to-four year follow-up of a controlled trial. *Psychosomatic Medicine, 41,* 229-242.

Reissman, F. & Scribner, S. (1965). The underutilization of mental health services by workers and low income groups: Cause and cures. *American Journal of Psychiatry, 121,* 798-801.

Rene, A.A. (1987). Racial differences in mortality: Blacks and Whites. In W. Jones & M. Rice (Eds.), *Health care issues in Black America: Policies, problems, and prospects* (pp. 21-42). New York: Greenwood Press.

Rose, S.D. & Tolman, R. (1984). *Leader's guide to stress management.* University of Wisconsin-Madison: School of Social Work.

Rudov, M. & Santangelo, N. (1979). *Health services of minorities and low income groups.* (DHEW Public Health Service #HRA79-627). Washington, D.C.: Government Printing Office.

Schreiber, J.M. & Homiak, J.P. (1981). Mexican Americans. In A. Harwood (Ed.), *Ethnicity and medical care* (pp. 263-336). Cambridge, Mass.: Harvard University Press.

Smith, M. & Dejoie-Smith, M. (1981). Behavior therapy for non-white non-yavis clients. *Psychotherapy, 21,* 524-529.

Turner, S.M. & Jones, R.T. (1982). *Behavior modification in Black populations.* New York: Plenum Press.

Turner, S.M. (1982). Behavior modification and Black populations. In S.M. Turner & R.T. Jones (Eds.), *Behavior modification in Black populations* (pp. 1-20). New York: Plenum Press.

Vernon, S.W. & Roberts, R.E. (1982). Prevalence of treated and untreated psychiatric disorders in three ethnic groups. *Social Science in Medicine, 16*, 1575-1582.

Waltz, M. (1986a). Type A, social context, and adaptation to serious illness: A longitudinal investigation of the role of the family in recovery from myocardial infarction. In T.H. Schmidt, T.M. Dembroski & G. Blumcheon (Eds.), *Biological and psychological factors in cardiovascular disease* (pp. 594-613). Berlin: Springer-Verlag.

Waltz, M. (1986b). Marital context and post-infarction quality of life: Is it social support or something more? *Social Science and Medicine, 22*, 791-805.

Waltz, M., Badura, B., Pfaff, H. & Schott, T. (1988). Marriage and the psychological consequences of a heart attack: A longitudinal study of adaptation of chronic illness after three years. *Social Science in Medicine, 27*, 149-158.

Wells, R.A. (1982). *Planned short-term treatment.* New York: The Free Press.

Wheaton, B. (1980). The sociogenesis of psychological disorder: An attributional theory. *Journal of Health and Social Behavior, 21*, 100-124.

Wilson, W. & Calhoun, J. (1974). Behavior therapy and the minority client. *Psychotherapy: Theory, Research and Practice, 11*, 317-325.

Wing, S., Casper, M., Riggan, W., Hayes, C. & Tyroler, H.A. (1988). Socio-environmental characteristics associated with the onset of decline of ischemic heart disease mortality of the U.S. *American Journal of Public Health, 78*, 923-926.

Wolinsky, F.D. (1982). Racial differences in illness behavior. *Journal of Community Health, 8*, 87-101.

Support for Parents of Children with Cancer: The Value of Self-Help Groups

Barbara K. Chesney
Kathleen A. Rounds
Mark A. Chesler

SUMMARY. Self-help and mutual support groups play an important role in the spectrum of resources useful to parents of children with cancer. These groups can provide parents with opportunities to share their experiences with other parents in similar situations, to learn from and teach others, and to create a new social network. While much has been written about such groups, very little attention has focused on factors related to parents' evaluation of their group experience. This paper examines factors related to parents' perceptions of the value of self-help groups.

In an effort to respond to persons affected by chronic and serious illness, medical professionals have developed medical strategies and protocols which facilitate treatment and recovery. There is, however, a need for clinical strategies which also recognize the psychosocial problems related to diagnosis and treatment. Nowhere is this need more acute than in the case of childhood cancer—a life-threatening illness which affects the family as a whole, over a long period of time, and whose victims cannot realistically advocate for

Barbara K. Chesney, PhD, is affiliated with the Department of Sociology, Anthropology, and Social Work, University of Toledo, 2801 W. Bancroft Street, Toledo, OH 43606. Kathleen A. Rounds, MSW, PhD, is affiliated with the School of Social Work, University of North Carolina at Chapel Hill. Mark A. Chesler, PhD, is affiliated with the Department of Sociology, University of Michigan.
Correspondence may be addressed to Dr. Chesney at the above address.

119

themselves. Parents must, with the help of medical professionals, take the emotional as well as the physical health of their family and their ill child into consideration. Social workers can be especially instrumental in helping parents do this, and there are a variety of ways in which parents can help themselves and be helped by social work practitioners.

For many parents of children with cancer, the first experience with long-term stress begins with the diagnosis of their child. That diagnosis brings both immediate and long-term stressors to bear upon the entire family of the ill child (Chesler & Yoak, 1984). Such stressors can appear in a number of forms. Intellectual stressors will test a parent's need for information about the child's conditions, while instrumental stressors will add to the everyday demands of practical family life. The advent of a child's diagnosis can produce changes in and tests of key relationships in a parent's life, and thus interpersonal stressors result. Finally, the threat of their child's illness and potential death can produce emotional stressors as parents try to cope with this threat, and existential stressors as they grope to make some meaning out of the crisis. Different parents will react to these stressors in various ways, and the challenge for clinical practitioners is to understand the full range of logistic, emotional, social, and medical concerns parents have. They also need to be able to respond on an individual basis to each parent's needs for coping resources and support.

Some parents will choose to react privately to their child's diagnosis and treatment, deciding not to seek support from others in their social network. For these persons, the role of the clinician is clearly one of individualized support and caring. Other parents may choose to supplement the care they receive from the psychosocial staff with the support and resources they can receive from others in their social world—family members, friends, and neighbors. Still others may prefer the information, sharing, and problem-solving that can emerge from contact with a group of similarly affected parents, other parents of children with cancer.

It is the set of parents who choose, often with the encouragement and guidance of a health care professional, to utilize the resources of other parents in the same situation that is our primary focus in this paper. The process of self-help and mutual support often provides parents with valuable information, emotional sustenance, financial help, and support through shared experiences (Chesler & Yoak, 1984). This has proven true in other arenas, and is true in the case of childhood cancer.

When parents join with others to make the physical and mental health of their child and family a working agenda, medical practitioners may wonder if that agenda, and the role of self-help groups, will always be positive and facilitating. As parents work to empower themselves on behalf of their child, health care professionals may become concerned about excessive parental intervention, misinformation, and interference with institutional practice. The power and resources of mutual support may appear as barriers to the medical process and system (Belle-Isle & Conradt, 1979; Binger et al., 1969; King, 1980; Mantell, 1983; Rosenberg, 1984). In order for professionals to view self-help groups as personally supportive to parents, and as positive vehicles for preventing and easing conflict between patients and providers, professionals must be given the opportunity to view the beneficial side of parent support groups and the value of these groups to parents.

The aim of this paper is to expand on the view of self-help groups in pediatric oncology in a way that provides clinical social workers with identifiable indicators of the value of such groups to parents. What factors contribute positively to the value of the group for those persons who choose to cope and seek support through self-help groups? How can that perceived value be facilitated by clinical social workers? The following analyses attempt to provide some answers to these questions.

SAMPLE AND METHODS

The findings reported here are from a larger study of self-help and mutual support groups for parents of children with cancer. The Candlelighters Childhood Cancer Foundation national network of groups was the primary study population, but independently organized groups, many of them off-shoots of Candlelighters' activities, were also included. Fifty self-help or mutual support groups were identified from a larger pool of more than 300 such groups. This was not a random sample of groups, but an informed, convenience sample. Groups were chosen with a goal of obtaining a useful mix from rural and urban settings, from various types of medical centers, with varying leadership structures, and representative of geographical regions nationally.

Data were collected using three methods: group interviews, a group information form, and questionnaires distributed to individual group members. First, on-site group interviews were conducted with parents and professionals (separately) who were involved with the local group.[1] The purpose of these interviews was to collect information about group history, structure, leadership patterns, and activities. As a follow-up to these group interviews, a group information form was mailed to the contact person (in most cases the social worker or a key parent) to obtain more information on frequency of group activities. In addition, individual questionnaires were distributed to parents by the contact person and returned to the study staff directly.[2] These questionnaires included questions regarding parents' characteristics, perceptions of benefits and effectiveness, leadership roles of parents and professionals, and attendance by spouses. Data collection methods are described in more detail elsewhere (Yoak & Chesler, 1985).

A brief summary of selected characteristics of these 50 groups is displayed in Table 1. Nearly three-fourths of these groups were led by parents, either independently of or in shared collaboration with professionals. One-fourth (13/50) were led and directed by professionals themselves. Almost two-thirds had been in existence less than three years; and more than two-thirds included parents of deceased children. For slightly more than half of the groups, the contact person with the medical system was the social worker. At least half had 11-20 members attending meetings, although close to one-third had less than eleven members attending meetings.

The characteristics of people who responded to a questionnaire distributed to a sample of members include those presented in Table 2. These individuals were primarily white, female, and married. Over half reported their spouse as occasionally attending self-help group meetings, over two-thirds were parents of living children, and two-thirds of the parents had taken some type of leadership role in the groups. Over 80% of the members lived within twenty-five miles of the meeting site.

Table 1

Characteristics of Parent Self-Help Groups (N=50)

Characteristics	Number	Percent
Leadership Type		
Parent Led	26	52.0
Shared (Parent & Prof.)	11	22.0
Professional Led	13	26.0
Group Age		
0-2.9 yrs.	31	62.0
3-4.9 yrs.	14	28.0
5 + yrs.	5	10.0
Include Parents of Deceased Children		
Yes	35	70.0
No	15	30.0
Number Attending Meetings		
5-10	16	32.0
11-20	26	52.0
21-50	8	16.0
Number in Active Core		
2- 7	26	52.0
8-18	17	34.0
20-40	7	14.0
Meeting Location		
Treatment Center	26	52.0
Community	18	36.0
Homes	6	12.0
Contact Person with Medical Center		
None	6	12.0
Social Worker	26	52.0
Nurse	7	14.0
Doctor	6	12.0
Parent/Professional	4	8.0
Other	1	2.0
Referral Process		
Medical System at Diagnosis	30	60.0
Parent-Linking Referral	20	40.0

Table 2

Characteristics of Parent Self-Help Group Members (N=146)

Characteristic	Number	Percent
Gender		
Female	123	84.2
Male	23	15.8
Race		
White	129	97.2
Hispanic	3	2.1
Other	1	0.7
Marital Status		
Married	132	90.4
Single	1	0.7
Separated/Divorced	11	7.5
Widowed	2	1.4
Spouse Attends		
Yes	79	55.6
No	63	44.4
Child's Status		
Living	102	69.9
Deceased	44	30.1
Type of Cancer		
Leukemia	82	59.4
Brain/CNS	16	11.6
Lymphoma	12	8.7
Bone	9	6.5
Wilms Tumor	5	3.6
Connective Tissue Cancer	14	10.1
Parents' Leadership in Group Activities		
Have been a leader	96	66.7
Haven't been a leader	48	33.3
Distance to Group Meetings		
Less than 10 miles	60	41.4
10 to 25 miles	62	42.8
25 to 50 miles	12	8.3
More than 50 miles	11	7.6

For this analysis, we chose to examine factors that we believed would make a difference in the value of the group to the members. The factors selected were those considered theoretically potent in understanding the value of a support group to members, and that could be targeted for interventions by social workers. The conceptual framework presented in Figure 1 displays the dependent and independent variables. Independent variables are grouped into five categories: group structural characteristics, professional involvement, frequency of group activities, members' reports of the benefit from group activities, and parent characteristics.

Group structural characteristics that were examined included: the number of parents attending meetings, the number in the active core, the contact person with the medical center, and helpfulness of American Cancer Society (ACS) contacts. The number of parents attending meetings and the constant supply of new participants are factors critical to the growth and development of self-help groups (Lieberman et al., 1988). In addition, an active core of members is crucial for long-term stability and development (Hill & Gruner, 1973; Scher, 1973). They are the key links who pass on the group's legacy and traditions, and help new members to assimilate (Schopler & Galinsky, 1984). Since all such groups are at least somewhat dependent upon the local medical system and community resource base (for referrals, for legitimacy, for financial and other resources), we also sought to assess the nature of their contact with the medical system and the role of the American Cancer Society representatives.

The exact form that professional involvement does or should take in self-help groups has been of interest both to professionals and to group members (Toseland, 1982). Professionals seem to function in a number of roles in groups: leader, therapist, consultant, liaison, referral source, and logistics manager. The analyses presented here examined whether the frequency of professional involvement in these various roles has an effect on the value of the group to members. The literature suggests that the type and frequency of professional involvement may influence the structure as well as the focus of the group. For example, Yoak and Chesler (1985) examined leadership patterns in self-help groups and found that professionally-led groups were smaller, did not as often involve parents of

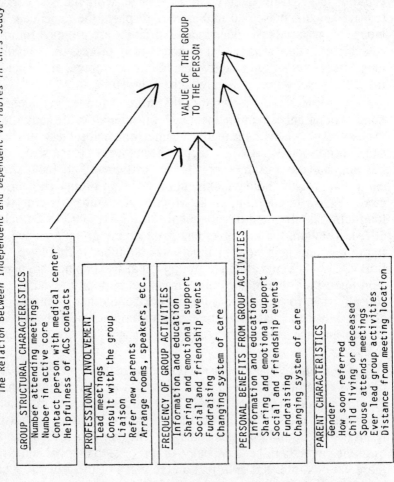

FIGURE 1

The Relation Between Independent and Dependent Variables in this Study

VALUE OF THE GROUP
TO THE PERSON

GROUP STRUCTURAL CHARACTERISTICS
    Number attending meetings
    Number in active core
    Contact person with medical center
    Helpfulness of ACS contacts

PROFESSIONAL INVOLVEMENT
    Lead meetings
    Consult with the group
    Liaison
    Refer new parents
    Arrange rooms, speakers, etc.

FREQUENCY OF GROUP ACTIVITIES
    Information and education
    Sharing and emotional support
    Social and friendship events
    Fundraising
    Changing system of care

PERSONAL BENEFITS FROM GROUP ACTIVITIES
    Information and education
    Sharing and emotional support
    Social and friendship events
    Fundraising
    Changing system of care

PARENT CHARACTERISTICS
    Gender
    How soon referred
    Child living or deceased
    Spouse attends meetings
    Ever lead group activities
    Distance from meeting location

deceased children, and stressed emotional support activities even to the exclusion of some other activities such as fundraising, engaged in by member-led groups. Supportive therapy often is the primary mode of activity in groups led by professionals. Professionals who serve as consultants do not directly lead the group, but may help parents establish a group by making referrals, training leaders, providing information and guidance on organizational matters, acting as facilitators and sponsors, understanding and intervening in particular problems, and identifying community resources to alleviate problems (Lurie & Shulman, 1983; Toseland & Hacker, 1982; Yoak & Chesler, 1985). Another professional role, that of liaison between the group and the medical center, may include legitimizing the group to other medical professionals in order to reduce professional fear of the group, encouraging support and referrals, and helping the group communicate with and perhaps influence the medical care system. Referring new members is another important way that professionals can support and legitimize self-help groups (Toseland & Hacker, 1982). Managing meeting logistics, another very common professional role, includes tasks such as scheduling meeting rooms, arranging for speakers, posting or mailing meeting notices, etc.

Work by Chesler and Yoak (1983) suggests that parent self-help groups primarily focus on five different kinds of activities to help members cope with the stressors associated with the experience of childhood cancer. These activities include the following:

1. *Information and Education*, e.g., presentations by medical staff on aspects of cancer and treatment, information on how to get hospital services, talks on how to deal with problems;
2. *Sharing and Emotional Support*, e.g., group discussions of parents' feelings, exchange of experiences, giving and getting support;
3. *Social and Friendship*, e.g., parties for families, special events for children, recreational programs, picnics and potlucks;
4. *Fundraising*, e.g., working on events or programs to raise money, finding sponsors or donors;
5. *Making Changes in the System of Care*, e.g., meeting with the

staff to suggest improvements, taking action on parents' complaints, working with schools to meet children's needs.

For the purpose of these analyses measures of both the frequency of each group activity and the amount of benefit attributed to the activity were used.

Finally, selected parent characteristics were included in the analyses. These characteristics are ones which clinicians and group leaders can influence or which other research has suggested as important: gender, length of time between diagnosis and referral to group, child's status (living or deceased), spouse attendance, parent participation in leadership, and distance from meeting location. We believed that the group would be of more value to parents who were female and who had higher educational status, because substantial prior research suggests that members of these population groups are most likely to participate actively—and presumably to benefit from—self-help groups (Gartner & Riessman, 1984; Lieberman & Borman, 1979).

We also assumed that parents who are referred to the group sooner after diagnosis would be more likely to attend and to benefit from the group than would parents referred at a later period of time, because the stress parents experience, and thus their need for the group's resources and activities, appears to be highest immediately at and after diagnosis (Chesler & Barbarin, 1987). On the other hand, Chesler, Barbarin, and Lebo-Stein (1984) suggest that parents are immobilized at this period of time, and are more likely to find the group of value some time (six months to one year) after diagnosis, when they have begun to adjust to the shock and to scan the environment for supportive resources. Prior research has also found child's status (living or deceased) to be an indicator of parent participation and perceived benefit (Chesler & Chesney, 1988).

We assumed that parents whose spouses attended meetings with them would find the group of greater value because they had responded as a total family, with their intimate support system committed and intact. Spouses who did not attend, especially if they were resistant to the idea of public sharing of feelings and problems, may have resented a spouse's attendance and made participation and benefit even more difficult to sustain. We expected parents who were involved in leadership roles in the groups to value the groups more highly because they should feel greater ownership or investment, either as a cause or effect of their estimation of its positive value. And, finally, we assumed that parents living nearer to the group's meeting location would value the groups more highly because they would find it easier to participate in meetings and activities than would parents who had to travel longer distances (Chesler, Barbarin, & Lebo-Stein, 1984).

The dependent variable in these analyses is a continuous measure of the value of the group to each individual, based on a closed-ended assessment of the overall effectiveness of the group currently, and a closed-ended report of the current level of importance of the group to the individual member. The higher the score on this dependent variable, the higher the level of the individual's perception of the self-help group's value to him/her personally. This measure of self-help group value attempts to incorporate both a judgement of group effectiveness and a report of current group importance.

One-way analyses of variance were conducted to examine and identify both the variables and the variable clusters that seemed to be associated with members' ratings of the value of the group. Table 3 presents the results from the analyses based on the members' responses (n = 146) to the individual questionnaire. Responses to open-ended questions or to the group interviews, which asked why parents thought the groups were effective or ineffective, also inform the interpretations of the findings.

RESULTS

Group Structural Characteristics

A number of group structural characteristics emerged as potential determinants of the value a self-help group can have for its individual members. The lowest group value was reported by members of groups where the primary contact person with the medical system was a physician. Persons in groups with larger numbers of individuals attending group meetings tended to report a higher overall group value to them personally, although this finding is not statistically significant. Persons in groups with the smallest active parent core reported the lowest group value. This finding is reinforced by

Table 3

Value of Self-Help Groups by Selected Factors

Factors	Value of Group F-statistic
Group Structural Characteristics	
# Attending meetings (140)	1.99
# In active core (140)	6.22**
Contact person with medical center (140)	2.97**
ACS contact (140)	.92
Professional Involvement	
Lead meetings (116)	.95
Consult between group and medical center (118)	3.11*
Liaison between medical center and group (111)	2.37*
Refer new parents (117)	.53
Arrange rooms, etc. (111)	.82
Frequency of Group Activities	
Information/education (140)	2.17
Sharing/emotional support (140)	.10
Social (140)	1.86
Fundraising (140)	1.95
Changing the system of care (140)	.72
Personal Benefits from Activities	
Information/education (117)	2.67*
Sharing/emotional support (128)	2.89*
Social (124)	1.75
Fundraising (118)	6.96**
Changing the system of care (114)	4.80**
Parent Characteristics	
Gender (140)	.078
How soon referred (121)	.47
Child living or deceased (140)	.29
Spouse attends (137)	2.09
Ever lead activities (139)	.34
Distance from meetings (139)	.91

$* \ p < .05$
$** \ p < .01$
N's are in parentheses

the qualitative data, which mention an active, involved core as more vital to overall perceived group value than attendance, per se. As one parent noted, "the core parents care about other parents and are trying to stress support." The level of helpfulness of the American Cancer Society (ACS) to the group did not make a significant difference in the value of the self-help group to parents.

Professional Involvement

Potential targets for intervention and correlates of group value were also revealed by analyses of characteristics of professionals' involvement with the self-help groups. Parents in groups where professionals more frequently consult with parents and act as liaisons with the medical center reported higher levels of group value. In contrast, the frequency with which professionals handle meeting logistics (e.g., get rooms, arrange speakers), lead meetings, and refer patients does not make a significant difference in reported group value. Thus, professionals' consulting and liaison work, rather than leading or arranging group functions, makes a positive contribution to the way in which individual members value the group in general. A quote from a parent illustrates the importance of a professional's facilitative role:

> As soon as your child is diagnosed, the social worker is right there to let you know and help out with all the benefits that the group has, like an apartment, and many things for the child to be entertained with.

Frequency of Group Activities

The various group activities included: information and education, sharing and emotional support, fundraising, social events, and changing the system of care. The data in Table 3 indicate that the frequency with which a group provided various types of these activities does not relate significantly to the value members attributed to the group. The frequency of informational/educational activities approaches significance in this relationship, but does not achieve it. These findings suggest that something beyond the frequent (or infrequent) provision of programs themselves generates value for members.

Personal Benefits from Group Activities

While the focus of these analyses is a measure of overall personal value of the group, it is assumed that personal value incorporates some general perception of the benefit of group activities. Specific categories of group activities were examined in terms of the degree to which parents' reported level of benefit from the activities related to the value of the group for them. The group was valued more highly by those members who reported the most benefit from informational/educational, fundraising, emotional sharing, and change work activities. An example of the benefits of these activities is provided by four parents:

> We need more medical experts to speak to us and to ask questions of.
>
> To be able to talk to people and learn that your problems are not something out of the ordinary.
>
> Resources — drug bank, gas mileage, apartment, food, toys, libraries . . . our services.
>
> As a group we really got the doctors to listen — parents could then be in with their kids for bone marrows.

However, perceptions of high benefits of social events did not lead to a sense of high group value. Members appeared to separate the informational gains and deep emotional sharing that occurred at group meetings from group sponsored social functions and parties. The latter events are common in most groups, are valuable and fun in and of themselves, and often help groups reach new members, but they do not contribute to the value parents assign to the group.

Parent Characteristics

We examined a number of parent characteristics and found that the extent to which parents value the group is not affected by various logistic and experience factors. Neither the meeting site nor the distance of the meeting from parents' residence appears to affect perceived group value. Similarly, parents' history as leaders, how soon they were referred to the group after diagnosis, and their spouse's attendance record do not significantly impact upon the overall value of the group for them. In fact, not even parents' gender or whether their children were living or deceased emerged as significant correlates of perceived group value. These results indicate that group characteristics, not selected parent characteristics, are associated with the value members place on the group. This finding suggests that a great deal of the potential for improving the value of the group for parents lies with interventions conducted at the group level.

DISCUSSION AND IMPLICATIONS FOR PRACTICE

Social workers can play a key role in supporting the development and growth of self-help groups and in helping to improve their value for parents. The results of this study suggest several guidelines for practice related to developing and maintaining an active group core, clarifying appropriate professional involvement, and aiding in planning activities that are of maximum benefit to parents.

Establishing and maintaining an active core depends upon (1) social workers and members developing and maintaining an effective recruitment and referral system that channels new members into the group; and (2) members finding a meaningful role in the group, feeling some ownership for the group, and sharing responsibilities and leadership. Because familiarity with self-help groups has been found to be a major predictor of whether or not social workers make referrals, a precursor to developing a referral system is for social workers to increase their awareness and understanding of self-help groups by attending meetings and meeting with group leaders (Toseland & Hacker, 1985). Social workers can improve the effectiveness of a recruitment and referral system by presenting the group to other professionals as a resource to parents, by encouraging professionals to support the group by referring parents, and by ensuring that the group has visibility and legitimacy in the medical center. Group members can work toward increasing and maintaining new membership by developing a system to contact all new parents directly and by ensuring that new members do not find it difficult to enter and attend a well-established group (Galinsky & Schopler, 1987).

Galinsky and Schopler (1987) discuss strategies for helping new group members quickly assimilate to open-ended groups and become functioning members: include older members sponsoring new members, phone and transport new members to meetings, and provide an orientation to new members when they begin attending meetings. Social workers who consult with members and leaders on how to run a group (e.g., running meetings, dividing tasks and rewards, recognizing service) can facilitate this process in ways that increase parents' sense of ownership. Anecdotal evidence suggests that an active core may be developed as a result of intense emotional bonding among a small number of parents who have shared important experiences with one another. Opportunities for such intimacy can be facilitated by social workers and, in turn, can facilitate the process of group development.

For many members this may be the first time they have belonged to a self-help group or any voluntary organization, and they may need guidance from others in order to experience how they can be helpful within the group while meeting their own needs. Many may lack leadership experience and may find feedback in how they function in this role to be helpful. Leadership training workshops jointly sponsored and attended by medical staff and by group members has been suggested as one way to develop and enhance leadership skills while increasing collaboration (Powell, 1987; Ayers & Chesler, 1987).

The results indicate that the type of professional involvement social workers undertake with self-help groups also makes a difference to parents. The roles of official leader and meeting manager are not as positively related to members' perceptions of the value of the group as are consultant and liaison roles. While skilled professionals can contribute to groups through their consultation on process issues, group members can provide valuable information to social workers through their consultation on the needs and concerns of parents, how parents support one another, and on ways to improve medical and psychosocial care. By developing the reciprocal nature of the consulting relationship, both professionals and group leaders can promote a more egalitarian and mutually empowering relationship (Powell, 1987).

If one of the tasks of people undergoing severe and chronic stress is to discover ways to "re-empower themselves" (Chesler & Chesney, 1988; Asch, 1984; Checkoway, 1985; Hatfield, 1981), leading their own group efforts certainly is a key part of this process. It is a way of contributing to others' welfare, as well as gaining aid for one's self. Professionals who usurp this self-assertive approach may frustrate an important part of the healing process; they may also stifle members' abilities to experience the gains of helping one another.

The findings from this study also suggest that social workers and nurses, rather than physicians, are the groups' most effective contact persons with the medical center. A major role of the social workers and nurses on the health care team is to provide psychosocial support to families and to help families negotiate the medical care system. Thus, social workers and nurses may have more time than physicians to devote to the group, especially if this task is included in their organizational role definition. Moreover, parents may be much more likely to share their concerns, particularly about quality of care, with social workers and nurses than with physicians. As a result, group members may feel that they can more effectively articulate their needs and engage in change activities directed at the medical system with social workers or nurses rather than with physicians.

The degree to which parents benefit from group activities makes a significant difference in how valuable the group is to them. This finding emphasizes that it is not simply the frequency of different activities that makes a difference, but the benefits parents derive from them. Thus, attention must be paid to the way activities are provided, not just to their provision, per se (e.g., parent or professional leadership of emotional sharing, purpose and style of fundraising, lecture or discussion format for informational events, etc.).

Parents enter self-help groups with varying needs based on many factors, such as their own coping strategies, background and experience with difficult situations, extent of existing social support, family situation, and experience with the medical center. These needs change as the child progresses through the phases of diagnosis, treatment, relapse, recovery or death. The fact that many parent self-help groups include parents of both living and deceased children (e.g., 70% of the groups in this study) illustrates the wide range of perspectives and needs that parents bring to these groups. In addition, the open-ended nature of self-help groups makes focusing on activities that meet the needs of the largest number of members more challenging—because the membership changes (Schopler & Galinsky, 1984).

Groups have developed a variety of strategies to meet the diverse needs of members (Chesler & Yoak, 1984; Schopler, Galinsky, & Alicke, 1985). One strategy is to focus on different purposes during alternating or rotating meetings and to have the various subgroups be responsible for the programming for their session. For example, the purpose of the first monthly session could be to share feelings or discuss emotional problems; the purpose for the second monthly session could be to organize social events such as holiday parties or child-centered activities. Another approach is to develop parallel structures, for example, separating a subgroup that conducts fundraising activities from a subgroup that meets to share feelings, or having partially separate meetings for parents of living children and parents of deceased children.

CONCLUSION

Working as partners in self-help groups, social workers and self-help group members can find ways to bring together both expert (professional) and experiential (parent) knowledge to strengthen the group, increase benefits for members, and potentially improve the medical system. If social workers are to enter into an effective collaborative relationship with self-help group members, many will need to increase their knowledge and skill in this area. The findings from a survey of 85 hospital social workers conducted by Black and Drachman (1985) found that respondents perceived a need for self-help groups and supported professional involvement in such groups; close to 90% of those surveyed approved of the role of consultant. However, many social workers noted that they lacked training and knowledge about support groups. Knowledge and education about self-help groups was found to be significantly associated with greater frequency of referral to the groups and perceived organizational support for the development of new groups. Almost half of these respondents indicated that that they would take a continuing education course on self-help groups. Social workers reported that they needed consultation skills, group process training, and group work skills relevant to their work with self-help groups.

The research reported in this paper indicates that parental responses verify these social workers' reports, and establishes an important agenda for social worker training. If social workers are to play truly helpful roles in self-help groups, as facilitators rather than therapists, as liaison agents and consultants rather than organizers and leaders, they will have to learn a great deal about group structures and processes, and about hospital and community dynamics. They also will need expanded exposure and information about the kinds of activities from which parents derive the greatest benefit. They will have to learn how to play an advocacy role with the medical system regarding publicizing the group and its activities, generating support for its legitimate functions, and gathering referrals. These new tasks and roles clearly call for in-service educational programs for social workers, as well as pre-service training, focusing on the realities of self-help group operations and activities.

NOTES

1. Of the approximately 378 persons interviewed for this study, 275 were parents (5-7 per group), 25 were social workers, 36 were nurses, 17 were physicians, and 16 were other health care professionals.

2. An average of 4 questionnaires per group were returned, representing half of the active core of the average group, and about 33% of the attendees at the average group meeting.

REFERENCES

Asch, A. (1984). The experience of disability: A challenge for psychology. *American Psychologist*, *39*, 529-536.

Ayers, T., & Chesler, M. (1987). Leading self-help groups: Report on workshop for leaders of childhood cancer support groups (Working Paper #351). Ann Arbor: University of Michigan, Center for Research on Social Organization.

Belle-Isle, J., & Conradt, B. (1979). Report of a discussion group for parents of children with leukemia. *Maternal-Child Nursing Journal*, *8*(1), 49-58.

Binger, C., Albin, A., Feuerstein, R., Kushner, J., Zoger, S., & Mikelsen, C. (1969). Childhood leukemia: Emotional impact on patient and family. *New England Journal of Medicine*, *280*, 414-418.

Black, R.B., & Drachman, D. (1985). Hospital social workers and self-help groups. *Health and Social Work*, *10*(2), 95-103.

Checkoway, B. (1985). Models for empowering citizens in human services. In *Patterns for Participation*. Wisconsin Association for Developmental Disabilities, Fall, 5-6.

Chesler, M.A., & Barbarin, O. (1986). *Childhood Cancer and the Family*. New York: Brunner/Mazel.

Chesler, M., Barbarin, O., & Lebo-Stein, J. (1984). Patterns of participation in a self-help group for parents of children with cancer. *Journal of Psychosocial Oncology*, *2*(3/4), 41-64.

Chesler, M., & Chesney, B. (1988). Self-help groups: Empowerment attitudes and behaviors of disabled or chronically ill persons. In H. Yuker (Ed.), *Attitudes Toward Persons with Disabilities*. New York: Springer, 230-247.

Chesler, M., & Yoak, M. (1983). The organization of self-help groups for families of children with cancer (Working Paper #285). Ann Arbor: University of Michigan, Center for Research on Social Organization.

Chesler, M., & Yoak, M. (1984). Self-help groups for parents of children with cancer. In H.B. Roback (Ed.), *Helping Patients and Their Families Cope with Medical Problems*. San Francisco: Jossey-Bass Publishers, 481-526.

Galinsky, M.J., & Schopler, J.H. (1987). Practitioners' views of assets and liabilities of open-ended groups. In J. Lassner, K. Powell, and E. Gennegan (Eds.), *Social Group Work: Competence and Values in Practice*. New York: The Haworth Press, 83-98.

Gartner, A., & Riessman, F. (1984). *The Self-Help Revolution*. New York: Human Sciences Press.

Hatfield, A. (1981). Self-help groups for families of the mentally ill. *Social Work*, *26*, 409-413.

Hill, W.F., & Gruner, L. (1973). A study of development in open and closed groups. *Small Group Behavior*, *4*(3), 355-381.

King, C. (1980, May-June). The self-help/self-care concept. *Nurse Practitioner*, pp. 34-5, 39, 46.

Lieberman, M.A. (1988). The role of self-help groups in helping patients and families cope with cancer. *CA-A Cancer Journal for Clinicians*, *38*(3), 162-175.

Lieberman, M.A., & Borman, L.D. (1979). *Self-help Groups for Coping with Crisis: Origins, Members, Processes, and Impact*. San Francisco: Jossey-Bass.

Lurie, A., & Shulman, L. (1983). The professional connection with self-help groups in health care settings. *Social Work in Health Care*, *8*(4), 69-77.

Mantell, J. (1983). Cancer patient visitation programs: A case for accountability. *Journal of Psychosocial Oncology*, *1*(1), 45-58.

Powell, T.J. (1987). *Self-Help Organizations and Professional Practice*. Silver Spring, MD: National Association of Social Workers.

Rosenberg, P. (1984). Support groups: A special therapeutic entity. *Small Group Behavior*, *15*(2), 173-186.

Scher, M. (1973). Observations in an aftercare group. *International Journal of Group Psychotherapy*, *23*(3), 322-337.

Schopler, J.H., & Galinsky, M.J. (1984). Meeting practice needs: Conceptualizing the open-ended group. *Social Work with Groups*, *7*, 3-21.

Schopler, J.H., Galinsky, M.J., & Alicke, M.D. (1985). Goals in social group work practice: Formulation, implementation, and evaluation. In M. Sundel, P. Glasser, R. Sarri, & R. Vinter (Eds.), *Individual Change Through Small Groups*. New York: Free Press, 140-158.

Toseland, R.W., & Hacker, L. (1982). Self-help groups and professional involvement, *Social Work*, *27*(4), 341-347.

Toseland, R.W., & Hacker, L. (1985). Social workers' use of self-help groups as a resource for clients, *Social Work*, *30*(3), 232-237.

Yoak, M., & Chesler, M. (1985). Alternative professional roles in health care delivery: Leadership patterns in self-help groups. *Journal of Applied Behavioral Science*, *21*, 427-444.

Yoak, M., Chesney, B.K., & Schwartz, N.H. (1985). Active roles in self-help groups for parents of children with cancer. *Children's Health Care*, *14*(1), 38-45.

The Crisis of the Forgotten Family:
A Single Session Group
in the ICU Waiting Room

Carolyn Holmes-Garrett

SUMMARY. This paper presents the problems encountered by relatives of hospital ICU patients. A review of the literature focuses on the nature and management of acute grief in a medical crisis setting. The interface between relatives and hospital staff around patient needs and family needs for information, guidance and support is also considered. A recommendation for group work intervention is made, and the role of the social worker as the appropriate agent of change in progress toward a hospital responsive to human need is discussed.

Sudden, life threatening illness, a serious accident, the critical exacerbation of a chronic condition; these are medical crises that develop without warning and throw families into tumult in an instant. A relative is carried to an ambulance and taken away. At the hospital, while the patient is being hooked up to monitoring and life sustaining machines behind closed doors the family tries to deal with the unreality alone in the anonymous glare of the ICU waiting room. The crisis causes disorganization; the family's physical and emotional homeostasis is drastically disturbed, and the situation demands solutions that are frequently outside their experience (Parad and Caplan, 1972). They are adrift in a strange and frightening predicament; the environment seems hostile, cold and alienating. The waiting room is probably uncomfortable and inadequate, and the staff are bustling and grave, busy saving lives. The family needs

Carolyn Holmes-Garrett, ACSW, MA, MSW, ATR, is affiliated with NYU, Spence-Chapin Services to Families and Children.

Correspondence may be addressed to Carolyn Holmes-Garrett at 243 W. 98 Street, New York, NY 10025.

emergency help too. In order to reestablish equilibrium, family members must recover adaptive resources and coping skills and be helped to deal with their emotional distress.

This paper will examine the phenomenon of acute grief and how it is expressed in the ICU setting. It will then address the needs of families of critically ill patients and the role of the social worker in this situation. Group work interventions that have been successfully used to provide support and reduce stress for ICU relatives will be described.

ACUTE GRIEF AND MOURNING IN A MEDICAL SETTING

The emotional health of the family is essential to rebuilding the health of the patient. Collaboration and cooperation are needed to reintegrate the ailing member into the family system (Leske, 1986; McGregor et al., 1981; Speedling, 1980). In order to intervene with the family, however, it is necessary to understand the process of acute grief, families' perceptions of their needs in a medical crisis and the most appropriate format for successful intervention.

Epperson (1977) describes six stages that must be negotiated; (1) anxiety, (2) denial, (3) anger, (4) remorse, (5) grief, and (6) reconciliation. The stages of grief can be compared to the responses to maternal separation found in children by Bowlby (1982). In this concept grief is seen as a variant of childhood separation anxiety following the disruption of an attachment. Children separated from their mothers for any substantial period protest, feel despairing and, finally, develop a defensive detachment to protect themselves from further painful affects. Families confronted with sudden, serious illness negotiate a similar process in their grief and mourning.

The family, according to Benoliel (1985), has the added burden of shifting relationships and social roles. Communication within the group can break down because of the illness and absence of the patient. An aunt may have to move in to care for the small children while their mother shuttles between home and hospital. Older children will have new and unwelcome responsibilities, at least for the duration of hospitalization. Existing or dormant family tensions are immediately exacerbated by the strain of adaptation which, in turn, is affected by cultural background, ethnicity and religious proscriptions. Financial strains and disrupted communication are often immediate problems which have had to be addressed before the actual grief work could begin.

NEEDS OF FAMILIES IN MEDICAL CRISIS

The management of sudden grief and mourning in a medical intensive care setting is a job no one wants. The staff are overworked and emotionally detached. They have not been trained to detect or deal with the problems of patients' families. Daley, a critical care nurse observed, "More often than not, the staff members in intensive care settings direct all of their energy toward saving the life of the patient . . ." (Daley, 1984, p. 234). The needs of family members are subordinated to those of the patient. In her study of the perceived immediate needs of ICU relatives, the desire for relief of anxiety, for information about the patient and for support and ventilation ranked high. They stated that they wanted ". . . the comfort and support of health professionals but perceived the professionals as being too busy to meet this need." Daley's view is that the well being of family members is the staff's responsibility and that this responsibility is not only underemphasized but most often overlooked. A follow-up study to Daley's work (Leske, 1986) stresses the family's need to feel that there is hope for recovery and to know that the patient is receiving the best care.

Daley feels that families are frequently too intimidated to speak to staff and thinks that time spent talking to them is time taken away from the patient. Their understanding of the patient's medical condition remains fragmented, and anxiety mounts. When family anxiety reaches an intolerable level and family members do venture to initiate contact the problems discussed are usually those perceived by the *staff* member to be important. This creates a wider gulf and can result in escalating stress for the family while the patient may, in fact, be improving.

Reaching Out to the Forgotten Families, Whose Job?

Many approaches to bridging the gap between staff/patient and family have been suggested. The liaison task generally falls to ICU nurses. They are increasingly asked to consider the patient's family as part of their primary care responsibility, instructed in ways to communicate more effectively with relatives and trained in crisis assessment (Massura, 1982).

Ambivalence, however, interferes with all ICU staff efforts to decrease the distance between themselves and the families of the patients they treat. The maintenance of a sense of distance is what protects staff from being drawn into the emotional drama that is the atmosphere of the ICU. It allows them to do their job in a competent, professional way in the face of relentless life and death crises. This emotional detachment and the intense pressure of their work interfere in a significant way with their availability to relatives in the waiting room. The social worker may be the professional best equipped to intercede with families and the ICU staff because of his/her position outside the unit structure; there are, however, problems of policy and role definition to be overcome.

Traditionally, the hospital social worker has ". . . played a subordinate role within the total complex . . . is a handmaiden to the physician . . . (and) is viewed and views herself [sic] essentially as a body mover, financial agent, and provider of prosthetic devices for individual patients" (Hallowitz, 1972, p. 90). Social service departments are often reluctant to offer clinical services in the domain of the physician where the psychiatrist is king of clinicians. Social workers perpetuate these conditions, safe in the knowledge that they are valued and secure on their own turf.

Doctors have the responsibility for life and death decisions and develop an authoritative manner which is, in part, useful and appropriate and, in part, defensive. This is reinforced by the nursing staff and sanctioned by society in general and makes it difficult for other health professionals to challenge their authority or to assume a peer relationship. Social workers, however, because of their training understand the importance of ". . . psychological reactions and the social implications of (illness) related to patient recovery and rehabilitation, . . . the realistic problems faced by the patient and his family . . . and (gathering) information about the patient's customary way of coping with problem situations'' (Ezra, 1967, p. 278). A position just outside the medical hierarchy gives the social worker the latitude to assess the service delivery system of the ICU and to make recommendations for more aggressive social work intervention with the families of patients, provided he/she has the backing of the department.

ENTERING THE SYSTEM, THE SOCIAL WORKER AS CHANGE AGENT

Hallowitz (1972) advocates the social worker mounting an intensive campaign to become an indispensable member of the ICU team. This can be done by attending staff rounds and introducing the idea that the social worker is available to relieve physicians and nurses of some of their most burdensome and uncomfortable tasks: talking to relatives about impending death, taking a family history, providing basic information, relieving anxiety, providing support and helping relatives to become a positive force in patients' illnesses. Ezra (1969) notes that families from cultural and socioeconomic backgrounds that are different from the attending physicians' think that the doctor is too busy to talk to them or will not understand their concerns. Benoliel (1985) found that cultural differences also alter the definitions of illness and the appropriate treatment for it. The specific cultural meaning of treatment can lead a family to seek help outside the medical system or to refuse to follow a prescribed medical regimen. Hispanic families, for example, will sometimes ignore prescribed psychotropic medication and take a psychotic family member to a spiritualist instead.

Social workers have a comprehensive grasp of the psychological, socioeconomic and cultural components of individual and family case management. This fact should be emphasized to the ICU staff in a specific plan designed to augment services to families, reduce pressure on staff and contribute to overall patient care. A format for periodic staff sessions to discuss difficulties, air grievances and improve inter-staff communication can be included in the plan. The social worker, as the purveyor of these services, must provide convincing evidence to the staff of group work and interviewing skills, comprehensive understanding of cultural differences, family systems, and psychological components of the grief process and knowledge of institutional organizational strategies.

SKILLS NEEDED FOR WORKING
WITH MEDICAL CRISIS FAMILIES

There are specific, interpersonal skills and degrees of self-knowledge required of the social worker in the ICU waiting room. A critical medical condition and the resulting anxiety and grief are extremely stressful for patients' families. The unprepared worker can be overwhelmed by the intensity of pain and the needs that are being expressed or, often, denied.

Besides familiarity with the process of grief and bereavement and a knowledge of crisis intervention, family and group work, the social worker must have a high degree of self-awareness. Working through one's own feelings about separation and loss allows for a more open attitude to the experiences of others and the ability to deal with the painful affects that constantly surface. Zisook and Shuchter (1986) note that coping with great emotional pain taxes the limits of the therapist's empathy. This is particularly true when facilitating the expression of a family's grief. Social workers must be given permission to ventilate their feelings and be assured that it is normal to feel as they do. In addition, reality testing and the acceptance of guilt and anger demand constant monitoring of the worker's own responses.

As someone outside the ICU system, the social worker becomes the repository for the staff's denied anxiety and anguish as well and must be able to understand and deal with these transference (and possible countertransference) issues when they arise. Obviously, a thorough grounding in psychology is needed along with the ability to absorb a great deal of strong emotion. Added to this list are secure interviewing skills, assertiveness and a knowledge of cultural differences in the grief process. Puerto Rican families, for example, often come en masse to the ICU waiting room and remain throughout the crisis with several members sleeping and eating there at all times while others take turns keeping things going at home. They talk and laugh and tell stories to keep their spirits up. A second generation Irish-American family, on the other hand, may tend to grieve quietly and in isolation.

THE SINGLE SESSION HOSPITAL GROUP

The family is a natural group. This suggests that its needs for support, encouragement and reaffirmation in a crisis could effectively be addressed in a group format. Literature on the use of group work in the ICU is sparse, but the single session group has been used in a variety of hospital settings. These groups are frequently task oriented and led by nurses (Bohannan-Reed et al., 1983) or hospital volunteers (Hodovanic et al., 1984). One single session waiting room group for diabetics had as its focus ". . . the development of a mutual aid system and support network in the natural setting of the waiting room" (Rotholz, 1985, p. 144). An ICU waiting room group run by two social work students (Bloom and Lynch, 1979) concentrated primarily on the dissemination of information. They found that information and education helped to reduce stress among the families in the group and that this format afforded the most productive use of the limited time available. Perry and Schwartz (1985) suggest that much can be accomplished in one meeting if the worker is experienced and directive and can facilitate maximum participation in the minimum amount of time. One-time members can benefit from a group if they learn a new coping skill, have some questions answered, or find support from an unexpected source.

The main problems faced by anyone trying to develop a group in a hospital, according to Robinovitch and Ransohoff (1981, p. 62)

> . . . are all related to institutional and professional power and territory. The territory is patient care. The power is the authority, sanction and control to propose the idea, negotiate its official acceptance, provide leadership to the group and to the staff in order to influence participant recruitment.

For these reasons it is absolutely essential to make a comprehensive presentation of the group protocol to the medical staff and to enlist their support. Resistance stems from a lack of familiarity with the group work modality in hospital treatment and from an unwillingness to change established routine. Attention to underlying problems of staff resistance to change and to incursion into their territory can clear the way for the introduction of the single session group into the ICU setting.

AN ICU WAITING ROOM GROUP

In 1985 an ICU waiting room group was developed in a municipal, teaching hospital in New York City. This ICU is extremely active and tension laden and at full census most of the time. The nurses and an attending physician are the only permanent staff. Because of the hospital's teaching function there is a constant rotation of medical, social work and psychology students. This provides further uncertainty and confusion.

Relatives of gravely ill patients wait for news and opportunities to visit in a small, narrow, cramped room with two rows of cold plastic chairs as the only furniture. There is a pay phone at the end of the room farthest from the open door, and patients from the medical ward, often trailing IV poles, use the room to make calls and to smoke, because their waiting room is frequently locked to keep out squatters and junkies from the street. The only visitors' bathroom on the floor is at the other end of the small room. The physical set-up is far from ideal. There is no way to close a group to prevent leaking boundaries. The heavy chairs are arranged in two rows along the walls and cannot be moved because of their size and weight. A chair must be brought in from the hall and placed in the middle of the rows at the end nearest the door, to block intrusion and discourage members from leaving a group session. Attention in the Intensive Care Unit is focused on the critically ill patients and relatives are, for the most part, ignored by the staff and wait in silence with their hopes, fears, anxieties and questions. Some pace the corridors outside the waiting room, and others make repeated trips to the first floor coffee shop.

The hospital social work department felt a strong need for a group to support and inform these family members in crisis, in order to help alleviate their anxiety and increase their availability to critically ill relatives. The group modality was chosen because this population has in common a very significant and galvanizing life crisis. It was thought that an opportunity to experience the universality of their dilemma through the sharing of problems, fears and questions would be more beneficial than individual interviews. It would also be more efficient, as more clients could be serviced at each contact. Because the author had group and crisis experience she was designated to organize and lead the group. This decision represented a progressive attitude toward patient care. At the time (1985), although five other major hospitals in New York City had perceived the need for group support in the ICU, none was currently sponsoring one.

In order to prepare the ground work for the group, contacts were made with the medical staff. Head nurses, staff nurses, an attending psychiatrist and medical residents were approached for opinions, ideas, support, and psychological validity from the medical quarter. A detailed protocol for the group was presented at medical rounds. The plan was received enthusiastically by the ICU staff who felt that they did not have the time or resources to deal with the neglected relatives and were willing to give the group a try. The group was announced by placing posters specifically aimed at the target population in the waiting room describing the purpose and time of the meetings.

The communities served by the hospital are ethnically mixed, with a large concentration of Irish-Americans and Italian-Americans living close by. Spread throughout the catchment area are an increasing number of Blacks and Puerto Ricans. The Italian and Irish-Americans are at the top of the social ladder, having been in the area the longest. They are mostly working class people with strong family and peer group ties that have been established over several generations. They speak the language, understand the local culture and are adept at finding and using available social service resources.

Blacks and Hispanics are the most frequent patients hospital-wide. Hispanics are the most disadvantaged segment of this population, with the most barriers to supportive services, including language and lack of familiarity with the dominant culture. Together with Blacks, who often face discrimination, they have the highest incidence of critical medical problems. A review of ICU records suggested that the waiting room sessions would draw primarily from Blacks and Hispanics. In fact, the weekly groups, which met for an hour to an hour and one half for a year, were generally composed of Blacks and Hispanics and Irish-Americans.

Purpose

The purpose of this group was to provide support and information for the relatives. In some cases admission to the ICU had come after months or years of serious illness, and one or more family members had been primary caretakers. In other cases a sudden heart attack had thrown the family into turmoil which they were ill equipped to handle. In all cases the relatives were being called upon to behave heroically in a grave crisis which severely tried their coping skills. For relatives of terminally ill patients the focus was on taking the first step in dealing with imminent loss. All families were helped to face their fears and anxieties and to cope with hospital procedures.

The social worker's goals were: (1) to modify the family-patient-hospital system in order to provide support and information; (2) to provide an outlet for the verbalization of worries about a serious health crisis or the possible death of a relative; (3) to help group members gain strength from each other; (4) to facilitate getting in touch with and expressing painful affects; (5) to create a network for mutual support; and (6) to help members to solve immediate problems in the group and in the wider environment. The leader's role in the group was to facilitate participation, provide support, model behavior, encourage interaction and supply information about hospital procedures.

Implementation and Ongoing Evaluation

All families in the waiting room, no matter what their ethnicity or the patient's prognosis, were dealing with the same crisis, a critically ill family member, and the same institution, the hospital. These were very important factors in the development of the group, because they created a sense of common emergency and, therefore, unity which allowed members to skip or condense the usual preliminary stages such as approach-avoidance, power struggle and differentiation that take place in long term groups (Yalom, 1975). Families were influenced by the emergent nature of their situation and were emotionally amenable to group sharing. Anxiety about the critically ill relative and fear and ignorance of hospital procedures from visiting hours to bill paying were common to all, no matter how many days they had already spent in the waiting room. The social worker facilitated intra-family and group communication and helped members to support each other.

Group members' primary needs were basic: care and feeding. Everyday lives had been disrupted, they were in an unrelenting state of anxiety, and the energy drain was great. Their need for nurturance was clearly evident in each meeting as they responded to a declaration of concern for them and their physical and emotional health. The fundamental need for emotional feeding was another important factor in mobilizing each group. It helped to keep members in the room in spite of disruptions and distractions and facilitated the condensed but discernible movement of the group through its developmental stages in every session.

Process

At the beginning of each "meeting" the goal of the leader was to make a group from the assembled visitors as quickly as possible, to encourage the verbalization of fears, anxieties and concerns and to provide emotional support. She introduced herself as a hospital social worker who was there to help with any problems "members" might have. She then mentioned a range of concrete problems (visiting hours, getting information from staff, location of the coffee shop) and suggested that families might have some other worries as well. The nature of these worries was intentionally left vague in order to elicit members' own associations.

At first, the goals of the group "members" were to be left alone and to avoid engaging in any interaction with the worker. They were surprised and not delighted to know that they were suddenly part of a group. They had not come to the waiting room for that purpose, and they perceived the social worker's presence as an intrusion. Sometimes one or two walked out. Frequently, having entire families present at meetings made the work of the group easier because family members were usually willing to talk to each other. The initial group resistance to talking with a collection of strangers was circumvented by this primary cohesion. If there were lone relatives waiting along with a family the willingness of the family to participate was often enough to pull the stranger into the group. The capacity to use the group experience seemed to be directly related to the strong motivation to get some support and nurturance in a period of great stress, once support was identified as the major purpose of the meeting.

Content

Group content was determined by the shared crisis. The need for empathic understanding was a constant theme. At the beginning of each session members were withholding and suspicious of an intrusion into their territory. At this point the worker always wondered how it could possibly turn around. Within minutes, however, after some gentle questioning by the leader about the nature of the relatives' illness, length of stay in the ICU and prognosis and some additional, tentative queries about their own feelings, members relaxed their guard and began to relate to the worker and to each other. The group identified family and individual networks and clarified ways in which members could ask for and receive help in this crisis. The need to verbalize fears and reminisce about patients' healthier days were common to all group members. It was the leader's job to encourage the cathartic release and exchange of this material, as well as to listen and express empathy. She also had to assess family systems and try to strengthen the weaker members without injuring the dominant ones. By promoting an atmosphere of caring and sharing she helped group members to provide each other with the nurturance they sought. The needs of individuals and the group as a whole were met in this exchange.

There were discernible patterns of interaction related primarily to ethnicity. The Hispanic families tended to be louder, more spontaneous in their interactions and affective expression, and to talk over and through each other. There was jockeying for position as one family member vied with another for the role of spokesperson. In the Italian and Irish families the hierarchy was clearer, and it developed along age and sex lines. The eldest son spoke for everyone present. If there were two families in the group, one Irish and one Hispanic they tended to talk only among themselves unless the worker could forge a bridge across which they could communicate with the other family. This usually could be done by identifying fears and questions common to all and encouraging one family to share their experiences with the other. The different families did not recognize the specific cultural and ethnic gaps between them, but there was a sense of guardedness and discomfort that had to be dispelled.

Mutual aid was one of the corner stones of the ICU group. It was evident as members sustained eye contact with each other and nodded in consent and support as one of their number recounted a poignant vignette or shared a secret fear that was identified as common to all. Doubts about staff competence and fears about approaching the doctors with questions surfaced frequently. At one meeting an Irish woman sparked group participation with the harrowing tale of her husband's arrival at the hospital by sanitation truck. Members also exchanged their experiences with social service agencies and gave tips about home health care. Their allegiance grew from intra-family to intra-group to extra-group in the time span of a single session. The following excerpt illustrates the rapid and telescoped development of a group session. It began with the members sitting in isolation, refusing to be a group. Links were finally forged through individual interviews, and members shared fears and anxieties, gave each other empathic support which fostered the development of self-control and, eventually, began to establish tentative networks. These could be continued outside the group.

Group Excerpt

Group members: Mrs. C. and her friend, Mrs. D. (Irish-Americans. Mr. C. had suffered a heart attack that morning). Mr. M. and his daughter, Ms. M. (Also Irish-American. Mrs. M. had been hospitalized for a heart attack and advanced cancer). Mrs. L., her stepbrother, Mr. R. and his wife (Hispanic. Mrs. L.'s and Mr. R.'s mother had also had a heart attack that morning).

After introducing herself the author explained that she was from the social work department and was here to help out in any way that she could, answering questions, providing information. She added that she felt that everyone was busy taking care of the critically ill patients, and that the relatives were often ignored. This usually helped people to start talking. This day it did not. They all looked guarded, and there was no interaction. After some awkward moments of silence, couples began talking to each other in low tones. The worker asked if anyone had any questions, if they all knew who their doctors were and if they knew the nurses' names. No. She offered to get them. She asked if anyone was having any problems getting information. No. She began to interview individual members. The others listened. She tried to establish herself as sympathetic, concerned, friendly, knowledgeable. She listened closely to what each member said and reflected the feelings expressed.

Everyone followed each interview carefully. The leader began to try to make connections between those who had obvious things in common, a relative with cardiac complications, Irish heritage. This worked. The Irish women asked each other tentative questions. Mr. R. said he had recently recovered from a heart attack. He looked quite healthy. This was reassuring to the others. However, he smoked constantly, denied being upset and denied that there was any reason for real concern. "Got to think positive," he said. He frequently changed the subject to the superiority of women and cited his stepmother's strength and good constitution as an example. Anxiety broke through his defenses several times, and he cried briefly. The women tried to calm him and told him he must stop smoking, but he was unresponsive. He seemed at risk for losing control, so the worker tried to reinforce their messages and, at the same time, to sympathize with how difficult it was to have someone very close to you so sick. This was useful for everyone. It articulated their pain in a low key way that allowed them to feel understood, but not overwhelmed.

The leader's role shifted from interviewing to listening and demonstrating empathy. Eventually she asked the group if they were all taking care of themselves during this crisis. This gave the members back a sense of autonomy and control around which they rallied. They began expressing concern for each other. Raising this issue also helped the relatives to feel cared for and lessened the feelings of loneliness and abandonment. They were having their own nurturance needs met. Questions were asked about visiting hours, monitoring and life sustaining machines, bedside protocol, local restaurants, insurance and the quality of care in the ICU.

The atmosphere in the group became more intimate and relaxed. Members shared information, and a network began to emerge. Mrs. L. and her stepbrother were able to reminisce about better times when their mother was well. The group ended with a feeling of catharsis (brief and fleeting but noticeable) and a sense of relief and renewal that had been achieved through the sharing of concerns, the expression of painful affects and the mastery of coping skills. The exchange of phone numbers indicated that a support network was likely to continue to operate after the group was over.

The six stages of grief enumerated by Epperson (1977) were condensed in this group as one stage merged into the next in rapid succession. This pattern was evident in all the single session waiting room groups. Following Daley's (1983) prescription for filling the needs of family members, the social worker focused on relieving anxiety, dispensing information, promoting the ventilation of affect and providing support. The reassurance and hope specified by Leske (1986) were fostered by answering questions about quality of care, life support machines, and patient monitoring.

It is clear from the excerpt and from the author's experience in the ICU that group work is a useful modality for this population. The ICU staff, at first wary of the intrusion, became ardent supporters of the relatives' group. In the session described, seven people from two very different ethnic backgrounds gained strength from each other and benefited, most of all from the mutual instillation of hope.

The single session group helps to bring together people in crisis who would otherwise remain isolated and neglected. It also serves to allay anxieties, provide comfort and understanding and encourage the development of coping skills. The group supplies members with an instant network for on-going support and reinforcement. The group configuration echoes the family configuration and can subtly influence the strengthening of family bonds. The group is beneficial to the ICU staff because it intervenes with patients' families to allow them to be more available to their critically ill relatives in ways that foster health and recovery or smooth the course of terminal illness. The hospital social worker, with a broad based knowledge of family and health systems, crisis intervention and the psychological, social and economic context is the professional best equipped to implement this service in the ICU.

REFERENCES

Benoliel, J., (1985). Loss and terminal illness. *Nursing Clinics of North America*, *20*(2), 439-448.

Bloom, N.D., & Lynch, J.G., (1979, August). Group work in a hospital waiting room. *Health and Social Work*, *4*(3), 49-63.

Bohanen-Reed, K., Dugan, D., & Huck, B., (1983, May/June). Staying human under stress: Stress reduction and emotional support in the critical care setting. *Critical Care Nurse*, *3*, 26-30.

Bowlby, J., (1982). Attachment and loss: Retrospect and prospect. *American Journal of Orthopsychiatry*, *52*(4), 664-678.

Daley, L., (1983). The perceived immediate needs of families with relatives in the intensive care setting. *Heart and Lung*, *12*(3), 231-237.

Epperson, M., (1977). Families in sudden crisis. *Social Work in Health Care*, *2*(3), 265-273.

Ezra, J., (1969). Casework in a coronary care unit. *Social Casework*, *50*, 276-281.

Hallowitz, E., (1972). Innovations in hospital social work. *Social Work*, *17*(4), 89-97.

Hodovanic, B. H., Reardon, D., Reese, W., & Hedges, B., (1984). Family crisis intervention program in the medical intensive care unit. *Heart and Lung*, *13*(3), 243-249.

Leske, J. S., (1986). Needs of relatives of critically ill patients; A follow-up. *Heart and Lung*, *15*(2), 190-193.

Massura, E. K., (1982). The view from both sides of intensive care. *Focus*, *9*(4), 3-5.

McGregor, E. A., Fuller, C., & Lee, M., (1981). Care and support for relatives in the ICU. *Nursing Times*, *6*(2), 1477-1478.

Parad, H. J., (Ed.). (1972). *Crisis intervention: Selected readings*. New York: Family Service Association of America.

Perry, J., & Schwartz, F. S., (1985, October), The application of the theory of single session groups to practice. Prepared for presentation at the Seventh Annual Symposium; The Advancement of Social Work With Groups. New Brunswick, N.J.

Robinovitch, A.E., & Ransohoff, M.E., (1981). Group work in general hospitals: Crisis intervention and politics. *Social Work with Groups*, *4*(3/4), 59-66.

Rotholz, T., (1985). The single session group: An innovative approach to the waiting room. *Social Work with Groups, 8*(2), 143-147.

Speedling, E. J., (1980). Social structure and social behavior in an intensive care unit: Patient-family perspectives. *Social Work in Health Care, 6*(2), 1-13.

Yalom, I., (1975). *The theory and practice of group psychotherapy.* New York: Basic Books, Inc.

Zisook, S., & Shuchter, S. R., (1986). The first years of widowhood. *Psychiatric Annals, 16*(5), 288-294.

Zisook, S., & Shuchter, S.R., (1986). Treatment of spousal bereavement: A multidimensional approach. *Psychiatric Annals, 16*(5), 295-309.

A Support Group for Burn Victims and Their Families

Judy A. Bauman
Greta L. James

SUMMARY. A rationale and description of a support group for burn victims and their families is presented. The open-ended group was designed and implemented to address the educational and emotional needs of participants. The sessions were organized and led by social workers with contributions from other disciplines. The support group appears to be an effective way to enhance coping for burn patients and their families. The needs for continued support for patients and families after discharge is also discussed.

Burn patients suffer from extreme pain, they often must cope with an altered appearance, and they frequently experience chronic emotional stress and other long term effects. The families of burn victims are also typically affected by some of the same emotional consequences. The major medical costs and lengthy separation from home and community are additional burdens for the burned-injured patient and family. Families usually are responsible for the care of victims after discharge and must endure long periods of recovery with them.

Consider, for example, the plight of the teenage mother whose 15-month-old baby was in a burn center. The young mother may have to deal with the anger of relatives who blame her for the burn and suffer an overwhelming sense of guilt because of the catastrophe. She has the additional stress associated with inadequate emotional and financial support while temporarily living away from home to be with her child. Her skills for coping may not be devel-

---

Judy A. Bauman, MSW, and Greta L. James, ACSW, are affiliated with the Department of Social Work, North Carolina Memorial Hospital, Chapel Hill, NC 27514.

159

oped at her stage of adolescence, and she can be overburdened by the unexpected tragedy. As Brodland and Andreasen (1974) note, under these conditions the young mother is still expected to function as a responsible parent, to take advantage of individual counseling, and to learn how to care for her burned child.

Unlike many other severe health problems, people rarely anticipate a serious burn, and therefore, most burn victims and their families are particularly ill-prepared to deal knowledgeably and emotionally with the catastrophe. As Goodstein (1985, p. 43) has observed, "Sudden onset with little or no warning, a lack of so-called premorbid 'worry time,' is a hallmark of catastrophes." It also is unlikely that the family will be prepared to cope with all that a burn injury entails. The family may find that the injury itself is repulsive, dirty, ugly, and has an odor. Acceptance of the injury may be particularly difficult when the burn is large, is located on the hands, face, or genitalia, the patient is extremely young or old, or the patient has pre-morbid psychological problems (Goodstein, 1985).

The conditions described above provoke innumerable comments and questions that must be addressed by social workers and other professionals responsible for the care of burn patients and their families.

"Which is worse — a first degree burn or a third degree burn?"

"Can I donate my skin if my son needs skin grafting?"

"If my mother lives for the next few days does that mean she will be okay?"

"I've never seen my dad cry."

"I won't be able to stand it if my child dies; I don't want to live if she doesn't make it."

"How could I have let this happen!"

"How will I ever pay for this?"

Family members need to confront these and many other questions, and they must consider the meaning of the accident and their emotions if they are to successfully begin to cope with the consequences. Burn victims and their families clearly have major informational and emotional needs. The medical staff must focus on the patient, which can leave the family alone to face the anxieties associated with the prospect of death, permanent deformity, and help-lessness. While the injured patient is progressing through the stages of resuscitation, recovery, and rehabilitation, the family also is moving along a similar path. Margaret Epperson (1977) identified six phases through which families in crisis might pass before they regain a homeostatic state: high anxiety, denial, anger, remorse, grief and reconciliation. Not all families will experience each phase, but their reactions, as well as those of the patients, need to be addressed.

The literature reveals the seriousness of a burn for the patient and family, and suggests that hospital support groups are a useful re-sponse (see, for example, Abramson, 1975; Brodland & And-reasen, 1974; Cahners, 1978; Rivlin, 1986; Weinberg & Miller, 1983). This paper describes a support group that was designed and implemented to respond to the needs of burn victims and their fam-ilies. It identifies major features of the group setting, objectives, development, structure, and implementation.

THE SUPPORT GROUP

Setting

The burn center where the group meets is a 21 bed unit in a large teaching hospital that provides treatment for burn victims through-out the state and occasionally from neighboring states. It has 11 intensive care unit beds, 10 intermediate care beds, a medical staff of 100, and a six-member psychosocial team. The Center admitted 212 patients in 1987. Of those patients, 166 were adults and 46 were children. Nineteen of the 212 patients died from their burns. Hospitalization averaged 18.8 days. All burn patients and their fam-ilies are eligible for the support group.

Goals, Objectives, and Strategy

Before the support group program began, information and sup-port for the relatives of burn victims were provided sporadically in response to individual initiatives by staff or family members. This situation was improved somewhat by the establishment of one-hour weekly meetings when staff provided information to groups of fam-ilies. These meetings did not directly address the emotional needs of the family, and they were cancelled when staff members perceived more urgent demands on their time.

As has been observed in the establishment of support groups in other situations (Bloom & Lynch, 1979), the group at the burn center evolved in part because a student social work intern was available to plan and implement it in collaboration with the social worker on the Center staff. The availability of a permanent social worker on the staff, and the commitment of all the burn center staff to the importance and success of the group, were essential to the group's establishment and viability. Other ingredients essential to the establishment of the support group were approval and support by the director of the Center, enthusiastic participation by staff members, and consultation from social work faculty.

The goal of the support group is to satisfy the informational and emotional needs of burn victims and their families in an efficient manner. Although the major focus is on family members, patients are included when they are well enough to attend. Objectives include providing specific education about burns and burn care, controlling rumors that permeate the waiting room, institutionalizing opportunities to ventilate, and providing psychosocial support. Specific objectives for family members focus on helping them better understand the victim's situation, and assisting in the return to the community. For patients, the objectives are to help them accept their current situation and to prepare them for return to their families and the community. The group is particularly conducive to instilling shared hope, an accurate perception of reality, and recognition that the lives of patients and families might be permanently altered. The social workers, within the group framework, demonstrate the interest and concern of the hospital staff and provide an open forum for questions and complaints. The group is viewed as an extension of, rather than as a substitute for, the individual relationships between patients, family members, and staff.

Formation and Development

Before implementing the group, information was gathered from 14 major burn centers in the United States that were similar in size. A letter was mailed to a social worker in each Center to obtain information about their support group programs. All 14 centers responded to the letter, and all had support groups. The features of some of those groups are reflected in our program.

To refine the program during its early stages of implementation, we also distributed questionnaires to participants at a meeting on psychosocial issues at the 1988 meeting of the American Burn Association in Seattle. The questionnaire asked about selected practices at their institutions, such as whether they had support groups for burn victims and their families, the features of the groups, and obstacles to successful implementation of support groups. The 18 respondents, from among approximately 27 participants, were social workers and other professionals from burn centers throughout the United States. The barriers to participation by burn victims and families included: (1) unavailable child care; (2) travel distance; (3) denial of the injury; (4) desire for insulation; and (5) discomfort in groups. The staff from other centers frequently cited the heavy demands of other responsibilities as a major barrier to the establishment of groups; the group had to function in the context of a busy intensive care unit. We attempted to solve the problems that were identified, but some people still were unable or unwilling to participate.

Leadership

The group is directed by social workers who coordinate activities and stimulate a milieu of group acceptance, belonging, and identification while assuring that the expertise of other professionals is shared with the patients and families as well.

Protocol

The support group meets once a week on the morning of a clinic day when no surgery is scheduled, a time most convenient for family members, patients, and staff. Meeting on a clinic day also allows participation by family members who accompany discharged patients when they return to the clinic for follow-up care. The support group meets the hour before family members visit the hospitalized burn patient, a time when relatives are particularly stressed because they are requested not to visit until tanking and dressing changes are completed.

A poster is placed in the waiting room each week to remind families about the meeting and to announce the topic. The social workers go to the waiting room to escort the family members to the meeting, thereby encouraging attendance and precluding confusion about the meeting location. The meetings are held in the Center conference room.

Attendance ranges from 3 to 15, with an average of 12 patients and family members attending each session. Patients are usually able to attend the group only toward the end of their hospitalization. Patients, family members, and staff members sit around a large table. The social workers begin by introducing themselves and describing the purpose of the meeting. They then invite the group members to introduce themselves, identify the patient with whom they are associated, and summarize the circumstances that precipitated the burn. The social workers emphasize the importance of families sharing their feelings and facilitate open and frank communication among members. The family members often indicate how long they have "lived" in the waiting room.

Refreshments, served after the introductions, help establish a cordial, informal, and non-threatening atmosphere that is conducive to open communication (Cahners, 1978). The social workers then announce the topic, introduce the speaker, and indicate how the speaker's professional skills relate to burn victims. The leaders also state that personal information will not be discussed in the group, and that questions about individual patients can be addressed confidentially after the meeting. Family members begin participating soon after the session begins because they readily recognize that they are with people who can empathize with them (Getzel, 1987).

In the first year of the support group, topics were organized to begin with information that is most salient at the time of admission and to proceed with information that becomes more meaningful as one nears recovery and discharge. The topics for each of the six sessions were addressed by speakers from different professions, as indicated: Session 1. Medical Concerns (Head Nurse); Session 2. Gross Motor Skills (Physical Therapist); Session 3. Fine Motor Skills (Occupational Therapist); Session 4. Faith in Crisis (Chaplain); Session 5. Discharge Planning (Social Worker); Session 6. Returning to Work or School (Rehabilitation Counselor).

The protocol for the support group was modified somewhat after the first year. The topics for each meeting, which had been decided a week before the meeting, are now decided two days before the session. Topic selection is based on identification of content that meets the immediate needs of the families, the current treatment phase of most family members, and concerns that are of immediate interest to the medical staff. The support group now meets two days after the regularly scheduled meeting of the burn center team, further facilitating timely suggestions from staff members. All topics from the first year were retained and the following new meeting topics were added: understanding burns and burn patients, visitation policy and procedure, coping with stress, skin grafting, adjustment to body image, and community education. Visual aids, such as slides and brochures, have also been added.

The topic schedule continues to be flexible so that issues that require immediate attention can be considered. For example, when the Center has several patients facing imminent death, the scheduled topic can be replaced by the session on Faith in Crisis so that the families can proceed together through the complex, painful, but normal and natural experience of grief (Taylor, 1988).

In addition to the regular speakers, other professionals, such as physicians, psychologists, and psychiatrists, participate as necessary. The presenters freely enter the sometimes serious, sometimes humorous, and always sensitive group interactions. A question and answer period concludes each meeting.

OPEN VERSUS CLOSE-ENDED GROUPS

Many professionals consider the closed group, characterized by stable membership, to be the preferred model. By necessity, however, most hospital-based support groups have constantly changing membership (Schopler & Galinsky, 1984). In a burn center, the turnover of patients requires an open-ended model where each session is viewed as discrete since members may be entering or leaving the group at any time. This model has been considered successful as well as practical in other environments (Alissi & Casper, 1985). The open-ended group is particularly appropriate for members who must cope with fluctuating emotions. An anxious new group member can respond positively to hearing what to expect from a person who has been a group member longer. Newcomers can also observe that others are functioning normally, and become hopeful that they too can achieve that level. Although close-ended groups are sometimes considered prerequisite to cohesion, strangers sharing similar crises can readily form bonds.

One session, then, could include the mother of a 15-month-old newly-admitted male, 60-year-old parents of a 32-year-old burn victim who is minimally invested in his rehabilitation program, mothers of two adolescents with non-threatening burns, and the wife of a patient who is going to die because of his burns. The next meeting might include some but not all of these members plus new members, and both old and new problems could be the foci of concern.

The open-ended format requires skillful and flexible leadership. The group leaders, in their efforts to provide continuity, must have the ability to respond to the emotional needs of both old and new group members, be able to assess the dynamic relationships among members, be capable of conveying warmth and understanding, and be able to maintain the group as a viable system of information and support.

SELECTED CASE STUDIES

The following examples suggest the impact of the support group in facilitating family adjustment and patient recovery. The first case illustrates how the group helped parents of an overly dependent son assist in their son's independence to assist his recovery. It also shows how the group helped the parents resolve feelings of guilt.

Case 1: The Family of K.C.

The parents of K.C. were very protective of their son who, at the time of his burn, resided with them even though he was 30 years old and gainfully employed.

From discussions in the support group, the parents began to recognize the need for K.C. to become independent. For example, the parents initially had to feed their son because his burn made it impossible for him to do it himself. However, his parents continued to assist him even when he became able. Several support group sessions were required for the parents to recognize why K.C. should feed himself even though it was painful and awkward for him. They eventually were proud that their son became able to complete the task as he rejected their attempts to help him.

The group also helped K.C.'s parents resolve the feelings of guilt often experienced by parents of burn victims, and to recognize that they were not responsible for being unable to relieve their son's pain and discomfort. Two months after discharge, K.C. moved into his own apartment for the first time and he and his family continue to have a mutually satisfactory relationship.

Case 2: The Family of Bobby Vee

A mother of a severely burned infant had few social and economic resources and low self-esteem. The group contributed to improvement in her self-confidence, social relationships, and childcare skills.

Ms. Jane Vee, a 20-year-old woman from rural North Carolina, is the mother of Bobby Vee. Bobby, a 21-month-old male, was admitted to the Center with a 54 percent body surface burn incurred while in the bathtub. The child had been deliberately burned by his father who was referred to protective service and not allowed to be in the Center.

In the beginning of Bobby's hospitalization, Ms. Vee was extremely passive and strongly influenced by Mr. Vee. She was frightened by the hospital environment and feared that her son might not survive. She had no social or financial support, and she realized that Bobby's father might be arrested and that she could lose custody of her son. Some staff members initially viewed her as an uninterested and possibly abusive parent.

Before Ms. Vee began participating in the support group, the social worker had been her sole source of emotional support and financial information. After attending several group sessions, Ms.

Vee began to smile, to talk freely with staff and other families, and to participate in the daily care of her son.

Ms. Vee received substantial support from other families in the group. She became involved in their activities and shared transportation with her roommate who was also a member of the group. It became apparent that she was a loving mother. She gained confidence by learning to care for her son and she took advantage of the group to discuss her feelings toward her son's father.

When Bobby was discharged after three months in the hospital, Ms. Vee was proud that she had become an important member of his treatment team. She had gained the self-esteem and efficacy required to deal with his return to the community.

SUPPORT GROUPS AFTER DISCHARGE

Discharge from the burn center is often followed by a long and difficult period of adjustment (Weinberg & Miller, 1983). A study by Wallace and Lees (1986) found frequent depression, anxiety, and alcoholism among discharged burn patients, and that most victims welcomed support groups. There are fewer organized support groups outside the hospital for burn victims and their families than there are for many other diseases and life-altering accidents. More attention to the social support of burn victims and their families could contribute to their adjustment and well-being following discharge (Weinberg & Miller, 1983).

Return to the community might be facilitated by public education programs, work-site interventions, and church efforts. School and job re-entry can be assisted by educating administrators about the burn victim and preparing others in their organizations for the patient's return. Support groups could be established locally to engage burn victims and their families in supportive therapy, and to advocate for community and occupational opportunity.

The importance of a support group in the hospital setting is magnified when sustained support is not readily available in the community. Adjustment by patients and families of burn victims will continue to be difficult in the hospital and in their homes. The support group described in this paper is a model to consider for addressing some of these needs.

REFERENCES

Abramson, M. (1975). Group treatment of families of burn-injured patients. *Social Casework, 56*, 235-241.

Alissi, A. S. & Casper, M. (1985). Time as a factor in social groupwork. *Social Work with Groups, 8*, 3-15.

Bloom, N. D. & Lynch, J. G. (1979). Group work in a hospital waiting room. *Health and Social Work, 4*, 49-63.

Brodland, G. A. & Andreasen, N. J. C. (1974). Adjustment problems of the family of the burn patient. *Social Casework, 55*, 13-18.

Cahners, S. S. (1978). Group meetings for families of burned children. *Health and Social Work, 3*, 165-172.

Epperson, M. M. (1977). Families in sudden crisis: process and intervention in a critical care center. *Social Work in Health Care, 2*, 265-273.

Getzel, G. S. (1986). Social work groups in health care settings: four emerging approaches. *Social Work in Health Care, 12*, 23-36.

Goodstein, R. K. (1985). Burns: an overview of clinical consequences affecting patient, staff, and family. *Comprehensive Psychiatry, 26*, 43-55.

Rivlin, E., Forshaw, A., Polowyj, G. & Woodruff, B. (1986). A multidisciplinary group approach to counselling the parents of burned children. *Burns, 12*, 479-483.

Schopler, J.H. & Galinsky, M.J. (1984). Meeting practice needs: conceptualizing the open-ended group. *Social Work with Groups, 7*, 3-21.

Taylor, B. (1988). Complexities of family grief in a burn unit: some social work dilemmas. *Burns, 14*, 46-48.

Wallace, L. M. & Lees, J. (1988). A psychological follow-up study of adult patients discharged from a British burn unit. *Burns, 14*, 39-45.

Weinberg, N. & Miller, N. J. (1983). Burn care: a social work perspective. *Health and Social Work, 8*, 97-106.

Groupwork in a Hospice Setting

Jack M. Richman

SUMMARY. Hospice has developed rapidly to become a major health care provider for those with a life threatening illness and their families. As part of their services, hospices offer several types of groups for their clients, volunteers and staff as well as social support groups for their own team members. This paper examines the functions of groupwork in hospice, focusing particularly on the use of hospice staff support groups. Research on the use of a group perspective and group methods in a hospice setting is presented.

Hospice has developed rapidly in this country to become a major health service provider for those with a life threatening illness and their families. Hospice, as a service delivery concept, made its way from London with the opening of the Connecticut Hospice in New Haven in 1974. Now only 15 years later, there are approximately 1568 hospices in this country (NHO, 1986). The services offered by hospice are currently a viable alternative to traditional health care for the terminally ill and services are included in and accepted by the federal government's Medicare Program. The major focus of hospice is on enhancing the quality of life for terminally ill clients and their families. Using an interdisciplinary model, hospice aids clients in maintaining control of their lives and in obtaining support from their families and health care providers.

The utilization of groupwork theory and practice is fundamental to the provision of hospice services. Hospice professionals must be conversant with group theory and practice because both the service system, i.e., the hospice team, and the primary unit of care, i.e., the client and family, function as groups. Whether the team exists

Jack M. Richman, PhD, is Assistant Professor, School of Social Work, University of North Carolina at Chapel Hill, Chapel Hill, NC.

as a free standing service system or is attached to a home health care agency or hospital, groups are a methodology used to enhance team functioning, volunteer training, and service delivery to clients. The hospice team operates as a multidisciplinary group to provide a matrix of services and support aimed at the physical, emotional, social, and spiritual needs of the patient and family. It therefore behooves hospice personnel to be knowledgeable and skillful in the management of groups for administrative and staff purposes as well as in serving the needs of clients.

This paper reports findings of a survey of the current use of various types of groups in hospice settings. It will further emphasize and focus on staff support groups for hospice teams whose goal is to serve as a buffer to vocational stress. Guidelines, based on survey results, a literature review, and practice experience, are suggested for establishing support groups.

SURVEY OF HOSPICE GROUPS

A stratified random sample telephone survey of hospices in North Carolina was conducted in March and April of 1988. Fifty of the state's hospices were selected from the 1986 *Guide to the Nation's Hospices* based on their location and the density of population area served. In this way, a statewide sample was created that included urban and rural settings, as well as various sized hospice teams. The final sample consisted of 44 (88% return) hospices; six hospices did not respond, could not be contacted, or were not fully operational at the time of the survey.

Each hospice representative, usually the director, was asked three questions designed to ascertain the current use of groupwork in the hospice: (1) What groups are you currently using in the provision of services to clients and families? (2) What groups are you currently using in the training, operation, and support of hospice volunteers and staff? (3) Who leads or conducts each group and how often do these groups meet?

Group utilization in hospice settings clustered into five areas as follows.

1. The Staff Meeting. All forty-four (100%) of the responding teams conducted staff meetings. These weekly meetings of paid staff were usually led by the nurse coordinator and were concerned with the daily operations of the clinical team, and the nature and needs of the clients served. These group meetings provided an opportunity for team members to share perspectives and informations.

Because hospice operates as a multidimensional team, there is often a blurring of professional roles. For example, the health aide may develop a close and intimate relationship with a particular client and family in the course of providing care services. When this is the case, the aide may become the primary confidant and support person who helps the client and family deal with many emotional issues related to the anticipated death. This role may generally be expected to be held by the social worker and/or nurse. However, because the staff functions as a multidisciplinary group, whoever can best provide services does so. For this reason hospice staff meetings tend to be more group oriented, more egalitarian, and less prescribed by traditional vocational roles and expectations than staff groups in more traditional settings.

II. The Interdisciplinary Team Meeting. All forty-four (100%) of the responding teams engaged in interdisciplinary team meetings. These meetings, generally held bi-monthly, include the entire paid staff who attend regular staff meetings, i.e., the Hospice Director, Nurses, Social Worker, Chaplain, Bereavement Coordinator, Health Aides, and Volunteer Coordinator plus the Medical Director and volunteers, i.e., all paid and non-paid team members currently involved with active hospice cases. The team meeting provides a mechanism for feedback and communication so that all individuals who are involved with a particular client and family can share information, concerns, and insights. This sharing provides the basis for patient family care plans regarding their medical, social, emotional, and spiritual needs.

III. The Bereavement Group. Bereavement groups are often facilitated by the team's Bereavement Care Coordinator or Chaplain. They meet monthly or bi-monthly, are free of charge, and open to members of the community who have experienced the death of a family member or significant other. Thirty-three (75%) of the responding hospice teams provided bereavement groups as part of service delivery and follow up care for families. The bereavement group may be time limited, e.g., 6-10 sessions, and then reconstituted to form a new group or it may function as an open-ended group with various members moving in and out of the group. Each of these models has positive and negative aspects regarding client access to group participation and leader ability to create a therapeutic group environment.[1] Whatever the specific design of the intervention, the use of groupwork for bereaved individuals provides the opportunity for clients to find and give support via ventilation, listening, and sharing of information regarding the bereavement process. It further allows the group members the opportunity to deal with their feelings of isolation, helplessness, and lack of control (Poss, 1981).

IV. The Volunteer Training and Support Group. Thirty (68%) of the responding hospice teams provided training and support groups for their volunteers. These group meetings, generally held once a month, offer education and training to volunteers as well as furnish recognition and social support for volunteers who deal with dying patients and their families. Examples of topics for volunteer training include: developing an understanding of the hospice philosophy, family dynamics and issues, legal aspects of death, AIDS, physical aspects of cancer and cancer treatment, grief and bereavement, and the role and responsibility of the hospice volunteer (Triangle Hospice Training Manual, 1987). Groups are facilitated by volunteer coordinators and hospice staff while other community professionals may supply some specific training programs.

V. The Staff Support Group. Seventeen (38.6%) of the responding hospice teams provided staff support groups and five additional hospices were planning them in the future. Support groups, generally held once a month, recognize and deal with the high levels of vocational stress under which hospice workers function.[2] These support groups are generally facilitated by an outside consultant. The group attempts to provide team support and act as a buffer to vocational stress.

These five areas of groupwork are currently being used by hospice teams in the provision of services to dying patients and their families. Groups provide clinical bereavement services for clients, provide needed training and social support for volunteers, function to provide the sharing of staff and patient information at staff and interdisciplinary team meetings and help reduce stress and burnout for team members.

There has been much written about the stress reduction function of social support groups and this concept has been applied to staff groups in health care settings including hospice. It is interesting to note that in the sample used in this research, team social support groups were currently active for 38.6% of the teams while the range for the other types of groups was from 68% to 100%. The social support groups for hospice teams is perhaps the newest use of groups in hospice settings. The following overview of the structure and function of support groups for hospice teams should provide an understanding of how group practice methods are being utilized to reduce hospice staff stress.

STAFF (CAREGIVER) SUPPORT GROUP

The belief that social support reduces stress has received widespread confirmation in the literature (Davis-Sacks, Jayaratne and Chess, 1985; Dean and Lin, 1977). Further, social support groups specifically designed for hospice workers are an accepted method for reducing or buffering the stress associated with the hospice as a work environment. This stress is a vocational reality because hospice care givers must constantly deal with dying patients, depressed family members, and equally stressed colleagues (Richman and Rosenfeld, 1987; Larson, 1986; Mor and Laliberte, 1985).

Vachon (1987) found that hospice workers may respond to stressors differently. Their responses include: conflict involving feelings of depression, grief, and guilt, dysfunctional interaction on the job and at home, and feelings of helplessness and insecurity. These worker responses can be dealt with in a variety of ways. One such method involves the use of social support. Osterweis, Solomon and Green (1984, p. 231) state: "By encouraging and structuring support for its staff, an institution demonstrates that it is aware of and concerned about the stress inherent in working with dying patients and their families." Many hospices recognize that vocationally related stressors exist and provide a staff support group for their team members. The majority of these support groups are held monthly and led by a chaplain or a counselor. Most often, the leader is not a team member but a consultant brought in specifically to conduct the staff support group. Although formal support groups may be preferred, support could also be obtained from other group experiences at work, e.g., staff meetings, informal groups, professional liaisons, or from non-work groups, e.g., family and friends or community groups.

There are a number of different models currently being utilized for providing staff support as a stress buffer. Larson (1986) adapted a training program called "Common Concern," designed to promote group cohesion and develop skills in communicating, building trust, giving empathy, and exploring options to meet the needs of a hospice and oncology staff support group. This twelve-tape series provides the basis for twelve structured group sessions specialized for hospice team support groups and coordinated by a team member. Examples of the topics covered are: motivation; purpose and goals of hospice and oncology workers; internal and external stressors; burnout and support; use of empathy, advice, and other communication skills; and suggestions for preventing burnout. Research regarding the use of this packaged material indicates it provides a high degree of team satisfaction (Larson, 1986).

Social support can be conceptualized "an exchange of resources between at least two individuals perceived by the provider or the recipient to be intended to enhance the well-being of the recipient" (Shumaker and Brownell, 1984, p. 13). When social support is used without clarification of the type of social support, it may be assumed that emotional and listening support are the forms provided (Albrecht and Adelman, 1984). Pines, Aronson and Kafry (1981) present an expanded version of social support and suggest that there are six distinct types of social support which individuals need to obtain from their environment.

1. *Listening.* Others who actively listen without giving advice or making judgments, with whom the joys of success as well as the frustration of failure may be shared.
2. *Technical Appreciation.* Others who acknowledge when a good piece of work is accomplished.
3. *Technical Challenge.* Others who are knowledgeable about an individual's work and can challenge, stretch, and encourage

the individual to achieve more, be more creative and excited about her or his work.

4. *Emotional Support*. Others who support an individual during an emotionally difficult time without necessarily agreeing with her or him.

5. *Emotional Challenge*. Others who challenge an individual to do her or his best to overcome obstacles and fulfill goals.

6. *Sharing Social Reality*. Others with similar priorities, values and perspectives who serve as reality "touchstones," with whom perceptions of the social context can be verified.

Richman and Rosenfeld (1987), utilizing the Pines et al. (1981) conceptual framework, conducted research about existing hospice support groups and found that while team members need to obtain all six types of social support from their environment, groups that were most effective in helping to reduce stress for hospice team members provided greater amounts of technical challenge, emotional challenge and shared social reality. It was also reported that effective stress buffering support groups in hospice de-emphasized listening support. These authors conclude that reflective listening ought not to be the goal of the support group as nonjudgmental listening may not offer the critical evaluations provided by technical challenge and emotional challenge support. Richman and Rosenfeld suggest that listening support be provided by people other than colleagues. Their research also suggest the importance of using an outside consultant who can help guide the group in providing its members with the most relevant types of social support. They also recommend encouraging members to establish networks external to the group where other types of social support can be provided.

The models proposed by both Larson (1986) and Richman and Rosenfeld (1987) recognize the connection of social support and hospice staff stress. They offer practitioners a set of guidelines from which they can gain direction and suggestions for group process when working with the hospice caregiver.

Using the hospice support group model proposed by Richman and Rosenfeld (1987), Richman (in press) suggests specific techniques which support groups might utilize to better provide the necessary types of social support.

Technical Challenge. (1) Have the group share the roles of each discipline or vocational area on the team with the team. This will allow each team member to better understand the professional roles and goals of their colleagues and thereby allow for more specific and relevant technical challenge support. (2) Encourage the involvement of the team members with their professional organizations on a local, state and national level. This involvement will present each team member the opportunity to discuss current vocational issues with similar professionals and obtain technical challenge.

Emotional Challenge. (1) Encourage discussion concerning death of patients and staff feelings towards patients and families. (2) Emphasize that team members cannot be all things to all clients. Discuss and process professional and personal goals, motivations, and limitations. These suggestions enable team members to connect emotionally with and stretch each other to meet and deal with the demands for hospice work.

Shared Social Reality. (1) Use and allow humor, even occasional humor that might be distasteful if taken out of context of caring professionals on a hospice team. (2) Encourage the team to share the unique demands and experiences of hospice work thereby allowing group validation. Sharing and relating experiences workers have had with clients and their families—the unusual and the difficult, the taxing and the emotionally intense—tend to reduce stress and set the experience into the reality of a work environment.

Listening (outside of the group). Encourage the team members to locate and participate in a formal support group in the community, e.g., Women's Center, or family or neighborhood networks. As noted earlier, while team members do provide listening support to each other while at work, support groups that were stress buffering tended to engage in technical challenge, emotional challenge, and shared social reality inside the support group, and obtain listening support from outside of the support group. Community networking allows team members to be listened to nonjudgmentally regarding hospice and non-hospice issues. They can shed their hospice role and be listened to as a nonhelping professional.

SCENARIO OF A SUPPORT GROUP

To provide an example of the use of hospice support groups, the following scenario is presented. It provides a snapshot of a hospice team social support group and demonstrates many of the requisite types of support as defined by Pines, Aronson, and Kafry (1981) while striving to emphasize those support elements of emotional challenge, technical challenge and shared social reality found to be critical by Richman and Rosenfeld (1987).

The Director, Patient Care Coordinator, Nurses, Social Worker, Chaplain, Health Aides, Volunteer Coordinator, Bereavement Coordinator, and Secretary seat themselves around the conference table. People are talking and drinking coffee. The leader, a consultant, asks the group how things are going at hospice. All are quiet—tension abounds. People look at the table, the ceiling, their hands—in what direction will the group move?

One Nurse speaks to the group about a patient's daughter who attempted suicide and the Nurse feels she should have noted the daughter's stress and anxiety level and foreseen the potential suicide attempt. The Nurse is upset and tears well up. The Social Worker and Health Aide suggest that many on the team missed the daughter's dangerous reaction to her father's rapid deterioration (emotional support) and state that it is important to deal with these issues (emotional challenge). The team allows the Nurse to express her feelings regarding being overwhelmed with the responsibility for people in her work and feeling out of control and incompetent (sharing social reality).

They support her and share their own similar experiences (shared social reality) and suggest that workers can do only limited amounts for their clients (technical support) and express that the Nurse is competent and does a good job (technical support and emotional support). The consultant probes for ways the other staff assess the family members' stability as the patient physically deteriorates and approaches death. Techniques and suggestions are made (technical challenge). The Nurse is back in control feeling accepted, supported and understood. She further has gained some techniques to implement in her next case.

The overall goal of staff support groups is to reduce staff stress and increase cohesion and feelings of professional competence. Achieving this goal will promote the effectiveness of the team in providing services to their clients and families. This approach does not attempt to analyze individual participants but seeks to allow each member to use the group to obtain the types of support she or he needs.

ESTABLISHING SOCIAL SUPPORT GROUPS

Establishing a support group for a hospice team begins by first recognizing that stress exists in hospice work environments and can and does affect the performance of the professional. Second, group implementation requires planning and support from the agency administration and staff.

To provide the appropriate setting for a stress buffering social support group one needs to help the agency administrators understand the unique nature of hospice work and the increased stress factors involved in this particular vocational environment. Hospice team members are dealing with a client population that generally dies within six months of the referral and intake of the case. At this point, the grieving process of the family and significant others become the prime concern. Therefore, workers go into client homes, providing a variety of services, establish intensive relationships and attend funerals within a relatively short period of time. Further, the nature of hospice work is such that staff must form caring, professional bonds with patients and their families and terminate these bonds relatively quickly. This forces staff to deal with their own grief for the loss of their clients on a continuous basis as well as face their own mortality and that of their family and children in each client's death (Schneider, 1987). While some of these issues are not wholly unique to hospice settings, the recurrent pattern of sustained intimacy, caring and involvement with clients over a period of months resulting in the assured outcome of death is very different from other health care environments.

Once the administration sees the value and need of a social support group for the team, some prerequisite conditions must be considered which have resource and policy implications. Issues such as staff time, allocation of resources, obtaining adequate space, and predicting and dealing with intra-agency staff relationships need to be examined.

Staff Time. Social support group meetings and staff meetings are not the same. Social support needs cannot be met in a typical weekly staff meeting (State, 1985). Support groups will be most effective if they meet bi-weekly or monthly and are separate times allocated for the sole purpose of a team support group. Staff time taken for a social support group is easily translated by administration into lost revenue due to non-patient and family contact.

Group Leadership. The support groups should be conducted by an outside (non-staff member) consultant. While leadership consultants generally become a resource commitment to the agency, making such a commitment has certain benefits. Using an outside leader for the group allows the staff to discuss personal concerns across professional lines as well as across lines of authority. It does not set one team member up as the leader which would prevent that individual from being a participating member of the group. It allows, for example, nursing staff to discuss the lack of pay for carrying the beeper on evenings and weekends with the Director; and the Social Worker to bring up concerns about not feeling competent to deal with the overwhelming grief of a family without feeling her supervisor will be making judgements concerning her performance. These status issues must be dealt with and worked on and, as trust develops, should dissipate to a tolerable level. An outside group leader enhances and provides some assurance of this status free environment as well as gives all members a chance to benefit from the group process.

Environment. The agency must provide adequate and comfortable space conducive to group participation and process. The area must provide staff with a degree of privacy so confidentiality can be guaranteed and further be a place where agency interruptions, e.g., telephone, client or volunteer needs, can be kept at a minimum.

Confidentiality. Confidentiality is a major issue in any group of this nature; however, some issues are unique to this situation. The outside consultant must ask the group to agree to some ground rules that guarantee that the Director and supervisors will participate as equals in the group and that they will not use material gained in the group sessions as the bases for vocational advancement. The support group will have difficulty functioning if this area of trust has not been dealt with. Another group rule is that the Director cannot call the consultant between group meetings to discuss individual and group issues. This discussion must take place in the group. However, the Director may call to evaluate the group's effectiveness or discuss the general stress level of the team due to an upcoming event such as a Medicare certification visit. Interactions between the Consultant and Director outside of the group must be handled carefully so as not to create the belief that they are in partnership separate from the group.

Intra-hospice Relationships. If the hospice is associated with a hospital or home health care agency, intra-unit jealousy may arise over concerns such as; hospice staff may be carrying a lighter case load (as measured in number of cases) and getting special consideration in relation to time and resources, e.g., to attend funerals and attend social support group meetings. These issues can be dealt with and discussed in the support group meetings and may at times include personnel from other health care units so they may understand the nature of hospice and perhaps see the need for some special consideration.

Ethical Implications. Requiring participation of hospice personnel in a social support group may cause increased stress and tension in some staff members. Open, honest communication of personal and work related issues may threaten some team members as they feel pressure to self-disclose in the support group. It is suggested that staff be expected to attend the support group regularly; however, the leader should stress confidentiality, privacy and trust and each group member's right to contribute or not, depending on comfort. Generally, resistive members will begin to engage with the group, to some extent, as trust develops and the group process proceeds.

Staff members need to understand the structure, function, and purpose of the support group. An understanding of the concept that obtaining social support from their colleagues can serve as a buffer for their vocational stresses may aid resistive members in joining with the group and allow the group as a whole to reach its desired goals and objectives.

CONCLUSION

Hospice teams use many groupwork methods and strategies to serve the needs of their clients as well as their own team members. Hospices use a team concept that focuses on support for families as the primary unit of care, values bereavement services, and recognizes the need for social support for hospice workers. The utilization and interest in providing a vocationally sponsored, stress buffering, social support group for teams are increasing in hospice agencies. Hospice staff work amidst a variety of stress chiefly stemming from dealing with the death of their clients and social support groups have been shown to be useful in combating these stresses. Hospice is an important innovation in health care delivery for those patients with a life threatening illness and their families. Social support groups can be a staff-saving method in maintaining a high quality of patient care.

NOTES

1. See Galinsky and Schopler, 1987, for a full discussion of this topic.
2. See *The Hospice Journal* special issue on stress and burnout among providers caring for the terminally ill and their families, Summer/Fall (2, 3) 1987.

BIBLIOGRAPHY

Albrecht, T.L. and Adelman, M.B. (1984). Social support and life stress: New directions for communication research. *Human Communication Research*, *11*, 3-32.
Davis-Sacks, M.L., Jayaratne, S. and Chess, W. (1985). A comparison of the effects of social support on the incidence of burnout. *Social Work*, *30*, 240-244.
Dean, A. and Lin, N. (1977). The stress buffering role of social support. *Journal of Nervous and Mental Disease*, *165*, 403-417.

184   GROUPS IN HEALTH CARE SETTINGS

Galinsky, M.J. and Schopler, J.H. (1987). Practitioners views of assets and liabil-
ities of opened ended groups. In J. Lassner, K. Powell and P. Linnegan (Eds.),
Social group work: Competence and values in practice (pp. 83-99). New
York: The Haworth Press.
Klein, A.F. (1972). *Effective groupwork*. New York: Associated Press.
Larson, D.G. (1986). Developing effective hospice staff support groups: Pilot test
of an innovative training program. *The Hospice Journal*, 2(2), 41-55.
Lattanzi, M.E. (1982). Hospice bereavement services: Creating networks of sup-
port. *Family and Community Health*, 5(3), 54-63.
Mor, V. and Laliberte, L. (1984). Burnout among hospice staff. *Health and So-
cial Work*, 9, 274-283.
National Hospice Organization. (1986). *The 1986 guide to the nation's hospices*.
Arlington, Virginia: National Hospice Organization.
National Hospice Organization. (1986). *Annual report to the membership*.
McLean, Virginia: National Hospice Organization.
Osterweis, M., Solomon, F. and Green, M. (Eds.). (1984). *Bereavement: Reac-
tions, consequences, and care*. Washington, D.C., National Academy Press.
Parks, C.M. (1972). Components of the reaction to loss of a limb, spouse or
home. *Journal of Psychosomatic Research*, 16, 343-350.
Parks, C.M. (1980). Bereavement counseling: Does it work? *British Medical
Journal*, 281, 3-6.
Pines, A.M., Aronson, E. and Kafry, D. (1981). *Burnout*. New York: Free Press.
Poss, S. (1981). *Towards death with dignity: Caring for dying people*. London:
George Allen and Unwin.
Richman, J.M. and Rosenfelf, L.B. (1987). Stress reduction for hospice workers:
A support group model. *The Hospice Journal*, 3(2/3), 205-221.
Richman, J.M. (In press). Social support for hospice teams: Strategies for effec-
tive groups. *Home Health Care Nurse*.
Schneider, J. (1987). Self-care: Challenges and rewards for hospice profession-
als. *The Hospice Journal*, 3(2/3), 255-276.
Shumaker, S.A. and Brownell, A. (1984). Toward a theory of social support:
Closing conceptual gaps. *Journal of Social Issues*, 40, 11-36.
Slate, E.C. (1985). Support systems are necessary for hospice readers and educa-
tors. *American Journal of Hospice Care*, 2(1), 11-12.
Vachon, M.L.S. (1987). Team stress in palliative/hospice care. *The Hospice
Journal*, 3(2/3), 75-103.